Empowering Caregivers Through Alzheimer's and Dementia:

Strategies for Families Living and Loving Beyond Memory Loss.

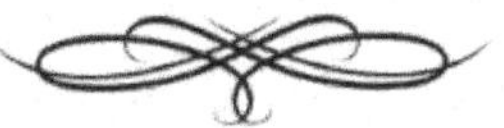

B.B. Goodings

Disclaimer

This book, "Empowering Caregivers Through Alzheimer's and Dementia: Strategies for Families Living and Loving Beyond Memory Loss," is intended to provide helpful and informative material on the subjects addressed. It is presented with the understanding that the author and publisher are not engaged in rendering medical, health, psychological, or any other kind of personal professional services in the book. If the reader requires personal medical, health, or other assistance or advice, a competent professional should be consulted.

The author and publisher specifically disclaim any responsibility for any liability, loss, or risk, personal or otherwise, which is incurred as a consequence, directly or indirectly, of the use and application of any of the contents of this book.

Important Note: The information in this book is based on research and personal experiences. While every effort has been made to ensure accuracy, the field of Alzheimer's and dementia care is constantly evolving. Therefore, readers should always check with professionals for the most current information and treatment options.

The author and publisher have listed the following key points to remember:

1. *Always consult with a healthcare professional for medical advice.*
2. *This book is a guide and not a substitute for professional medical care.*
3. *The experiences and strategies discussed may not apply to all situations.*

Foreword

As a physician who has dealt with Alzheimer's and dementia in my own family, I am both honored and privileged to write the foreword for this indispensable book, "Empowering Caregivers Through Alzheimer's and Dementia." This work is not only a beacon of knowledge but also a guiding light for caregivers and as well as dementia patients who are navigating the challenging journey of these conditions.

Alzheimer's and dementia are not just medical conditions; they are life-altering experiences that affect patients and their families profoundly. The emotional, physical, and psychological toll can be overwhelming. However, with the right knowledge, support, and resources, caregivers can transform their roles from mere caregivers to empowered advocates and compassionate companions.

This book serves as a comprehensive resource for both caregivers and those dealing with this disease, providing invaluable insights into the complexities of Alzheimer's and dementia. It offers practical advice, emotional support, and evidence-based strategies that caregivers can utilize to enhance the quality of life for their loved ones and themselves. From understanding the early signs of dementia to managing the later stages, each chapter is a treasure trove of information that addresses the diverse aspects of caregiving.

One of the most commendable aspects of this book is its emphasis on empowerment. Empowerment in caregiving is not just about having the knowledge; it's about cultivating resilience, fostering hope, and building a supportive community. The stories, tips, and guidance shared within these pages remind caregivers that they are not alone in this journey. There is a community of professionals, fellow caregivers, and organizations ready to support them every step of the way.

I wholeheartedly recommend "Empowering Caregivers Through Alzheimer's and Dementia" to anyone involved in the care of individuals with these conditions. It is more than a book; it is a lifeline, a source of strength, and a beacon of hope. May it inspire and guide you as you embark on this noble journey of caregiving.

Dr. Meredith C. Wills, DO

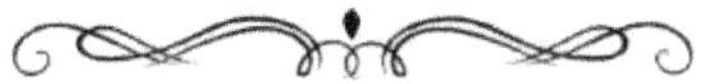

Dedication

I dedicate this book to the incredible caregivers and family members who selflessly and affectionately support those facing Alzheimer's and dementia, and to those individuals courageously confronting these challenges themselves. The journey can be a profound test of endurance – lengthy, draining, and deeply isolating.

I want you to know that there are individuals out there ready to lend a helping hand. I've written these words with the sincere intention of offering hope and valuable resources to all of you. Having personally navigated this journey within my own family, I intimately grasp the struggles involved, and my heart genuinely extends to each and every one of you.

By sharing these stories amd resources, I aim to not only acknowledge the difficulties but also to provide practical insights and support. Recognizing the emotional toll and the sometimes overwhelming nature of caring for those with Alzheimer's, this book is my attempt to be a source of encouragement, offering a lifeline to anyone grappling with the complex challenges of Alzheimer's and dementia care.

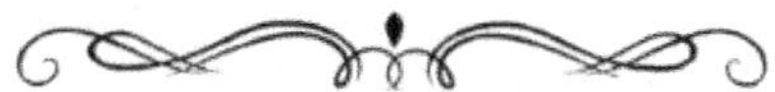

Contents

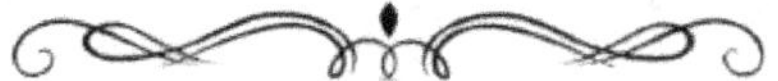

Introduction

American politician Brad Henry once said, *"Families are the compass that guides us. They are the inspiration to reach great heights and our comfort when we occasionally falter."* This sentiment captures the essence of the story I'm about to share.

Samantha and her family were much like any other. Sunday dinners, annual vacations, and surprise birthday parties marked the milestones in their lives. As time went on, the family noticed subtle changes in Grandma Mary. She'd forget where she left her glasses, sometimes even misplacing them in the fridge. Then, she began forgetting birthdays and eventually struggled to recognize familiar faces.

Mary's Alzheimer's diagnosis hit the family hard. Samantha grappled with a mixture of emotions - sadness, frustration, and often helplessness. Yet, amidst the challenges, she discovered that caregiving was not just about providing physical and emotional support. It was also about cherishing the shared moments and finding joy in the seemingly mundane. Learning about Alzheimer's and dementia became a mission for Samantha. She delved deep, wanting to provide the best care for Grandma Mary. She learned about the brain's functions, how Alzheimer's affects it, and the various treatment options available. More importantly, she discovered strategies to connect with her grandmother, even on challenging days.

One of Samantha's most treasured moments was when she played Mary's favorite song. Though Mary couldn't remember Samantha's name, she hummed along to the melody, her eyes lighting up with recognition. It was in these moments that Samantha realized that while memories might fade, emotions and feelings lingered.

While Samantha's journey was unique, her experiences resonated with many caregivers worldwide. Navigating the waters of Alzheimer's and dementia requires patience, love, and understanding. It's essential to remain informed and equipped with the right strategies. Being informed empowers caregivers to offer the best care possible, enhancing the patient's quality of life.

But it's not just about the patient. Caregivers, too, need care. It's a role that demands much, often leading to emotional and physical exhaustion. Balancing personal needs with caregiving responsibilities becomes crucial. Finding a support system, be it through family, friends, or support groups, can make all the difference.

Samantha's story isn't uncommon. Across the globe, countless families endure similar experiences, seeking understanding and support. This book aims to provide just that. From a deep understanding of Alzheimer's and dementia to practical caregiving techniques, we delve into various facets of these conditions.

While the medical aspects of Alzheimer's and dementia are vital, the emotional journey is equally important. As Samantha's story reveals, it's the little moments that matter. The spontaneous laughter, the shared song, or the brief moment of recognition are the moments that bring joy, offering solace in the midst of challenges.

Why This Book

"In the heart of every caregiver is a deep well of love, waiting to be poured out." - Unknown Author.

Being a caregiver to someone with Alzheimer's or dementia is no small task. But you're not alone. Many families find themselves in this situation. They often seek three things: knowledge, strategies, and emotional support. This book aims to provide all three.

Alzheimer's and dementia can be confusing. But with the proper knowledge, they don't have to be. The goal here is to make these conditions more understandable. This book is not about flooding you with medical jargon. It's about breaking things down in ways that make sense.

When we say knowledge, we mean comprehensive details. This book covers the causes, symptoms, and treatments of Alzheimer's and dementia. It's not just a surface glance. It dives deep. Yet, it remains accessible. Think of it as a well-guided tour through a maze. One step at a time, we'll navigate this together.

Now, knowledge is great. But what about action? That's where strategies come in. Every caregiver wants to do their best. They want their loved ones to have a good life. Yet, it can be hard to know what to do. This book offers practical tips. These are not abstract ideas. They are real-world actions that can make a difference.

Some strategies are simple. Others might need more effort. But each one is tested and proven. They come from the experiences of other caregivers, just like you. They've been where you are. They've faced the same challenges. And they've found ways to rise above.

However, the heart of caregiving is not just about tasks. It's also about emotions. As a caregiver, you might feel a mix of feelings. There could be love, hope, and joy. But there could also be stress, fatigue, and sadness. It's natural. It's human.

Emotional support is crucial. And that's a big part of this book. Interspersed with facts and strategies are stories. These are tales of real families facing Alzheimer's and dementia. They share their ups and downs, their triumphs and tears. These stories offer a glimpse into the lives of others. They show that even in tough times, there's hope.

Remember, every person's experience is unique. Yet, there are common threads that bind caregivers. By reading this book, you join a community. It's a group of people who care deeply and give their all. People who face challenges but never give up.

Prologue: A Glimpse into the Journey Ahead

"Alzheimer's and dementia are not just conditions of the mind; they touch the heart, soul, and very fabric of families."- Unknown Author.

Empowering caregivers is at the heart of our mission. We'll walk you through a comprehensive guide crafted specifically for families navigating the complexities of Alzheimer's and dementia. From deep dives into the science behind these conditions to touching personal narratives, we've got you covered.

The first chapter gives you a robust understanding of Alzheimer's and dementia. You'll learn about their differences, the science underpinning them, and how to recognize their early signs. We delve deep but always make sure the information is easy to grasp.

Diagnosis and treatment options come next. This chapter sheds light on the medical landscape surrounding these conditions. Real-life accounts peppered throughout give a human touch to the often clinical world of medical interventions. Beyond the traditional, we also explore alternative and complementary therapies that families have found beneficial.

Your role as a caregiver is invaluable. In the third chapter, you'll find stories of individuals just like you who stepped into this vital role. Learn from their challenges, their solutions, and their emotional journeys. This chapter also touches on the legal and financial aspects, offering guidance in these often overwhelming areas.

Maintaining connections with our loved ones as they journey through

Alzheimer's or dementia is paramount. Chapter four is dedicated to this. From personal stories of resilience to expert advice on effective communication, this chapter emphasizes the power of the human connection.

Next, we venture into creating a supportive environment for your loved ones. Learn about home modifications, the power of routines, and day-to-day activities that can make a world of difference.

Well-being isn't just about the mind. Chapter six delves into the pivotal roles of nutrition, physical health, and mindfulness. You'll learn how these elements synergize, fostering caregiver and patient well-being.

Chapters seven and eight bring more nuanced discussions to the table. These sections offer depth and insight, from transitioning to advanced care and hospice to navigating the intricate maze of legal and ethical considerations.

The impact on family dynamics forms the core of chapter nine. You'll read touching accounts from siblings, spouses, and even grandchildren who've taken on caregiving roles. These narratives highlight the far-reaching impacts of Alzheimer's and dementia on family relationships.

Lastly, we turn our gaze towards the future with hope in chapter ten. From the latest scientific advancements to inspiring tales of families building legacies, this chapter is a beacon of optimism.

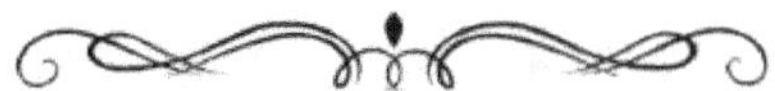

Chapter One
Understanding Alzheimer's and Dementia

"The first step toward change is awareness. The second step is acceptance." -
Nathaniel Branden.

At its core, understanding Alzheimer's and dementia starts with knowing what they are. Both are terms that refer to a group of symptoms which affect memory, thinking, and social constructs severely enough to interfere with daily life. But they aren't the same thing.

Alzheimer's is a specific disease, the most common cause of dementia. It's named after Dr. Alois Alzheimer, who first identified it in 1906. It's a progressive disease, which means it gets worse over time. It affects the areas of the brain that control thought, memory, and language. Over time, a person with Alzheimer's may have trouble remembering things, making decisions, and even carrying out basic tasks.

On the other hand, dementia is a general term. It describes symptoms that impact memory, everyday activities, and communication abilities. Alzheimer's is just one type of dementia. There are also other dementias, such as vascular dementia, Lewy body dementia, and frontotemporal dementia. Each type has different causes and may affect people in different ways.

While Alzheimer's disease makes up 60-80% of dementia cases, not everyone with dementia has Alzheimer's. It's like saying every square is a rectangle, but not every rectangle is a square.

Now, it's important to note that age is the most significant risk factor for both Alzheimer's and most types of dementia. While a normal part of aging, the risk of Alzheimer's and dementia increases significantly as you get older. They primarily affect older people but can also affect younger people in rare cases.

Early signs of both Alzheimer's and dementia can include mild forgetfulness, losing track of time, and getting lost in familiar places. But, Alzheimer's disease specifically may also present with mood changes such as increased confusion, fear, or suspicion.

Treatment for Alzheimer's and dementia varies. It can include medication, cognitive training, and therapy. Unfortunately, there's currently no cure for Alzheimer's, but there are treatments which can slow the worsening of symptoms and improve quality of life.

Each person with Alzheimer's or dementia has a unique experience. Symptoms and disease progression can vary widely. It's a challenging journey, not only for those diagnosed but also for their caregivers and loved ones.

Understanding the difference between Alzheimer's and dementia is vital. It allows for better management of the condition, more accurate expectations, and better caregiving strategies.

Remember, knowledge is power. The more you know about Alzheimer's and dementia, the better equipped you'll be to support your loved one through this experience. It's about loving and living beyond memory loss, providing the best care you can, and finding strength in the face of adversity.

The Magnitude of Alzheimer's and Dementia Prevalence

"Alzheimer's is relentless. Dementia is relentless. But so, too, are we." - Lisa Genova.

We start by setting the stage with some hard facts. Alzheimer's disease and dementia are not rare conditions. They touch the lives of millions across the globe. The World Health Organization reports that around 50 million people worldwide have dementia, and nearly 60% live in low to middle income countries. Every year, there are almost 10 million new cases.

The prevalence of Alzheimer's and dementia is significant and rapidly growing. Alzheimer's Disease International estimates that by 2050, over 152 million people will be living with dementia. That's roughly equivalent to the entire population of Russia, the world's biggest country. This staggering number underscores the urgent need for understanding and managing these conditions.

Let's delve deeper into the numbers. Alzheimer's disease is the now most common form of dementia, accounting for 60 to 70% of all dementia cases. The remaining cases are due to other conditions such as vascular dementia, mixed dementia, and Lewy body dementia, among others. These figures reveal that dementia is a wide-ranging term covering a variety of conditions, each with its unique challenges.

Age is a major risk factor for Alzheimer's and other forms of dementia. The Alzheimer's Association reports that one in 10 persons over the age of 65 has Alzheimer's dementia. After the age of 85, the risk of developing dementia from Alzheimer's nearly doubles. It is crucial to note that while dementia is more common in older people, it is not a normal part of aging. There is also a significant gender disparity in dementia prevalence.

Women are more likely than men to develop Alzheimer's and other forms of dementia. Nearly two-thirds of Americans with Alzheimer's are women. The reasons for this disparity are still under investigation. Still, some studies suggest a combination of biological, genetic, and lifestyle factors.

Unfortunately, dementia is underdiagnosed. According to the Alzheimer's Society, only about 50% of people living with dementia have a formal diagnosis. This means many people are living with dementia without knowing it, missing out on the support and treatment they need.

In the United States, Alzheimer's and dementia are a significant public health concern. The Centers for Disease Control and Prevention reports that in 2020, an estimated 5.8 million Americans aged 65 and older were living with Alzheimer's dementia. By 2060, this figure is projected to nearly triple to 14 million.

The economic impact of Alzheimer's and dementia is equally significant.

The total global cost of dementia was estimated to be $1 trillion in 2018, and that figure is expected to double by 2030. The costs include direct medical costs, social care, and informal care (care provided by family members and friends).

The prevalence of Alzheimer's and dementia underscores the urgent need for effective interventions, support for caregivers, and ongoing research into these conditions. It's a clarion call for us to understand these conditions better and strive to improve the lives of those affected.

The numbers also hold a promise. They remind us that if you are a caregiver for someone with Alzheimer's or dementia, you are not alone. Millions of families worldwide are walking the same path. There is a global community of caregivers, a network of people who understand the unique challenges, joys, and heartaches of caring for a loved one with dementia.

Neurological and Physiological Underpinnings Explained

"In the depth of every soul, there is a door that leads to healing." - Gerald G. Jampolsky.

As a caregiver, you might wonder what causes Alzheimer's and dementia. Let's untangle this puzzle. We'll begin with the brain. This organ is like a command center, controlling all our body functions. When changes occur in the brain, it can affect how we think, feel, and behave.

Now, imagine billions of nerve cells in the brain. These cells, or neurons, are the basic building blocks of the nervous system. They communicate with each other through signals. In Alzheimer's and dementia, these signals get disrupted. Why does this happen? It's due to a build-up of proteins in the brain. In Alzheimer's, these proteins form plaques and tangles. In other types of dementia, different proteins are involved.

These proteins disrupt the normal functioning of neurons. Over time, these neurons lose their ability to communicate. They eventually die, leading to brain shrinkage. This process happens slowly, over many years. It starts in the part of the brain responsible for memory. This is why memory loss is often the first symptom of these conditions.

But it's not just about proteins and neurons. There's more to this story. Factors like inflammation and oxidative stress also play a role. Inflammation is the body's response to injury. But when it becomes chronic, it can harm neurons. Oxidative stress, on the other hand, is an imbalance between free radicals and antioxidants in the body. Too many free radicals can damage neurons.

So, you see, Alzheimer's and dementia are complex conditions. They involve multiple processes in the brain. Understanding these processes can help us find new ways to manage these conditions. But remember, you're not alone in this journey. There are many resources available to help you navigate through these challenges.

Now, let's talk about the effects of these changes on the person. In the early stages, the person may start forgetting recent events. They may repeat questions or get lost in familiar places. As the disease progresses, they may struggle with ordinary tasks like cooking or paying bills. Their personality may also change. They may become anxious, depressed, or irritable.

Understanding these changes can help you provide better care. It can also help you cope with your own emotions. You might feel frustrated or sad when your loved one forgets your name. But remember, it's the disease, not the person. They're not doing it on purpose. It's just their brain trying to cope with the damage.

In the later stages, the person may need help with basic tasks like eating or bathing. They may also need help with speaking or understanding words. They might not recognize their family members. These changes can be hard to witness. But remember, your loved one is still there, even if they can't express it.

Caring for someone with Alzheimer's or dementia is not easy. It takes patience, understanding, and love. But it can also be rewarding. It can deepen your connection with your loved one. It can teach you about strength and resilience. And it can show you the power of love beyond words and memories.

Recognizing the Signs

"The beginning of all understanding is recognizing what is." - Socrates.

We often hear stories of people who, in hindsight, saw the signs but did not realize what they meant. Mary's mom, for example, was always so organized. So when she started forgetting where she placed her things,

Mary thought it was just part of aging. But it was more than that. It was one of the first signs of Alzheimer's.

Mark's dad was the life of the party. He loved social gatherings and never missed a family event. But slowly, he started withdrawing, often looking confused and lost in social settings. It wasn't just old age. It was the beginning of dementia.

These stories remind us that recognizing the signs is the first step. It's not about finding a reason to worry but about staying informed. Knowing what to look for can help you take early action and get the right help.

Alzheimer's and dementia often start subtly. Memory loss that disrupts daily life is a common early symptom. It's not just forgetting names or appointments but more significant issues like forgetting recent events or asking for the same information over and over.

Another sign is difficulty in completing familiar tasks. People with Alzheimer's may have trouble driving to a familiar location or remembering how to play their favorite game. They may also struggle with visual images and spatial relationships, particularly having trouble reading or judging distance.

People may have trouble following a conversation or finding the right words as the disease progresses. They may also start misplacing things, putting them in unusual places. They may even lose the ability to retrace their steps.

Recognizing these early signs can be a game-changer. It can lead to a quicker diagnosis, which opens up more treatment options. It allows for planning for the future and making legal and financial arrangements. It also allows the person with dementia to participate in decisions about their care and future.

Of course, every person is different. Not everyone will have the same symptoms or progress at the same rate. This is why consulting with healthcare professionals when you notice changes is essential.

You might think, "But these signs could also be a part of normal aging!" And you're right. It's not uncommon for people to forget things or get confused as they age. But when these symptoms become frequent and interfere with daily life, it's time to seek help.

In the case of Mary's mom, it was her persistent forgetfulness that led them to seek medical advice. They learned that her forgetfulness was not just a part of aging but a sign of Alzheimer's. For Mark's dad, it was his withdrawal from social events and his confusion in familiar settings that raised concerns. His diagnosis of dementia came as a shock, but it also brought clarity and guidance.

The journey of recognizing the signs is not easy. It's filled with uncertainty and worry. But remember, you're not alone. There are resources and support available to help you navigate this path. You have the power to make a difference in your loved one's life, and it starts with recognizing the signs.

Let's take a lesson from Mary and Mark's stories. If you start to notice changes in your loved one's memory, behavior, or abilities, don't ignore them. Seek help. It's the first step towards understanding, which is the first step towards better care.

Remember, Alzheimer's and dementia don't just affect the person diagnosed - they impact the entire family. By recognizing the signs early, you're not just helping your loved one - you're also helping yourself and your family. You're laying the groundwork for a plan, for support, and for hope.

Recognizing the signs is the first step, but not the only one. As you navigate this journey, remember to also take care of yourself. Caring for someone with Alzheimer's or dementia can be challenging, but you don't have to do it alone. Reach out, get support, and remember to take time for self-care.

Just like Mary and Mark, you, too, can navigate this journey with strength and grace. Recognizing the signs is just the beginning. With knowledge, support, and care, you can not only cope with Alzheimer's and dementia but also improve the quality of life for your loved one.

Common Symptoms and Their Impact on Daily Life

"Alzheimer's is not a part of getting older; it's a disease that affects our loved ones, slowly stealing their memories." This quote paints a stark picture of the reality we are dealing with. As a caregiver, your role is vital, and understanding the common symptoms of Alzheimer's and dementia is the first step toward effective caregiving.

Memory loss is one of the most common signs of Alzheimer's. It's more than simply forgetting where you placed your keys. It's about forgetting recent events, names, or faces. It's about asking the same questions repeatedly, even after they've been answered. This symptom significantly impacts daily life, making it hard for your loved one to carry out simple tasks.

Another symptom is confusion with time or place. It's not uncommon for someone with Alzheimer's to lose track of dates, seasons, and the passage of time. They might forget where they are or how they got there. This can disrupt daily routines and lead to frustration and anxiety.

Difficulties with words in speaking or writing also become apparent. They might have trouble joining a conversation, struggle with vocabulary, or repeat themselves. This can make social interactions challenging and potentially lead to isolation.

Alzheimer's and dementia can also lead to changes in mood and personality. Your loved one might become confused, suspicious, depressed, fearful, or anxious. They might get easily upset at home, work, with their friends, or when out of their comfort zone. These changes can strain relationships and make caregiving more challenging.

As these symptoms progress, they impact daily life in profound ways. Simple tasks like cooking, cleaning, or even dressing can become difficult. Social interactions may dwindle as communication becomes challenging.

The world can become a confusing, frightening place for your loved one.

Understanding these symptoms and their impact is a crucial step in your caregiving journey. It equips you with the knowledge to provide the best care possible, tailored to your loved one's unique needs. This understanding can also foster empathy, making navigating the emotional challenges of caregiving easier.

Keep in mind that every person with Alzheimer's or dementia is unique. The symptoms and their progression can vary significantly from person to person. It is important to stay patient and flexible and adapt your care strategies as needed. Always remember, you are not alone in this journey. A wealth of resources and support is available to aid you in this journey. Chapter Two will go into these options in much more depth.

The Importance of Early Diagnosis and Intervention

"Knowledge is power. Information is liberating. Education is the premise of progress, in every society, in every family." - Kofi Annan.

By now, you know that Alzheimer's and dementia are not easy foes. These are conditions that can turn your world upside down. But there's hope. One key weapon in our fight against these diseases is early diagnosis. Why? Because it allows us to take action. And action can make a world of difference.

When we catch Alzheimer's or dementia early, we can plan. We can start treatments that may slow the disease. We can make choices about care. We can even use the time to make memories and share stories. It's an opportunity to make the most of the time we have.

In the early stages of Alzheimer's and dementia, changes may seem minor. Forgetfulness. Trouble with routine tasks. Mood changes. These signs can be easy to miss. But they can also be the first clues to what's happening.

When we spot these signs, it's crucial to seek medical help. A doctor can run tests. They can ask questions. They can do a complete check-up. From this, they can make a diagnosis.

If the diagnosis is Alzheimer's or dementia, it's a tough blow. But an early diagnosis gives us power. It gives us options. It lets us plan for what's to come. It allows for early intervention.

Early intervention begins with a care plan. This is a roadmap for dealing with the disease. It's a guide for the journey ahead. A care plan can include medications, therapies, and strategies for day-to-day living.

Medications can help manage symptoms and slow the progress of the disease. They can help with memory loss, confusion, and mood changes. While they can't cure Alzheimer's or dementia, they can make living with these conditions a bit easier.

Therapies can also be a big help. These can include physical therapy, speech therapy, and cognitive therapy. These therapies can help maintain physical strength and mental function. They can also give caregivers tools to help manage the disease.

Strategies for day-to-day living are also a key part of early intervention. These can include tips for managing routines, creating a safe home, and dealing with challenging behaviors. It can also offer ways to keep your loved one engaged and active.

In addition to medical and practical support, early intervention can also offer emotional support. It can connect you with support groups, counseling, and resources. It can provide a community for people who understand what you're going through.

Early diagnosis and intervention can also offer a chance for your loved one to take part in clinical trials. These are studies of new treatments and therapies. They can offer hope for the future. While an early diagnosis of Alzheimer's or dementia is tough, it's also a chance. It's a chance to take action. It's a chance to plan. It's a chance to get the support you need.

Stages and Progression

"Understanding is the first step to acceptance, and only with acceptance can there be recovery." This insight from J.K. Rowling can help guide us as we explore the stages of Alzheimer's and dementia.

Alzheimer's and dementia progresses in stages. The path is not always straight. Each person's journey will be different. However, knowing the stages can help you understand what to expect.

The first stage is the "no cognitive decline" stage. At this point, the disease is not yet outwardly detectable. Memory and mental abilities are normal. Next comes the "very mild decline" stage. You may notice minor memory problems or lose things around the house. These changes are often mistaken for normal aging.

The "mild decline" stage follows. Friends and family start to notice memory and cognitive problems. Your loved one may need help remembering simple words or with tasks like balancing a bank account.

The "moderate decline" stage is next. Memory loss and confusion become more evident. People may forget details about their lives, feel moody, or have trouble dressing.

In the "moderately severe decline" stage, people may need help with daily tasks. They may not remember what day it is or their personal history.

The "severe decline" stage is challenging. People may have trouble recognizing family and friends. They may also have difficulty walking, talking, and swallowing.

Finally, the "very severe decline" stage is the final stage of Alzheimer's. Because of damage to the brain, people may lose the ability to communicate or move.

Case Studies

"Remember, we can't control the wind, but we can adjust the sails," Cora L. V. Hatch first stated it reflects the unpredictable nature of Alzheimer's and dementia and how we can adapt to the changes that occur. As a caregiver, understanding how symptoms progress is vital to providing the best care.

Alzheimer's and dementia are not one-size-fits-all diseases. Symptoms can vary from person to person, and the rate at which they progress also differs. Let's consider a few examples to illustrate this.

Consider the case of Mr. Johnson. When his family first noticed changes, they were subtle. He would forget where he put his car keys or miss a doctor's appointment. But over time, these memory lapses became more frequent. He started forgetting names and faces, even those of his close family members. This stage is often referred to as mild Alzheimer's.

As the disease progressed, Mr. Johnson started having difficulty completing familiar tasks. He found it hard to follow recipes, even though he used to be an excellent cook. He would become confused about where he was or what day it was. His family also noticed changes in his mood and personality. He became easily upset and suspicious. This stage is often referred to as moderate Alzheimer's.

In the late stage of Alzheimer's, Mr. Johnson needed round-the-clock care. He had difficulty communicating and became unaware of his surroundings. He also experienced physical changes, such as weight loss and difficulty walking. This case illustrates the progression of Alzheimer's, but remember that it can vary between individuals.

Another example is Mrs. Smith. She was diagnosed with vascular dementia after suffering a stroke. At first, her symptoms were primarily physical, such as weakness on one side of her body. But over time, she started experiencing cognitive changes. She had difficulty planning and organizing, and her memory also started to decline.

Unlike Alzheimer's, the progression of vascular dementia can be a bit unpredictable. Mrs. Smith had periods where her symptoms seemed to stabilize, followed by sudden declines after subsequent strokes. This illustrates how different types of dementia can have different progression patterns.

Lastly, let's look at the case of Mr. Rodriguez, who was diagnosed with Lewy body dementia. His first symptoms were not memory-related at all. Instead, he experienced visual hallucinations and changes in his sleep patterns. He also had movement symptoms similar to Parkinson's disease, such as a shuffling walk and tremors.

As his disease progressed, Mr. Rodriguez started experiencing cognitive symptoms. He had difficulty with attention and decision-making, and his memory also declined. His symptoms tended to fluctuate from day to day, which is a characteristic feature of Lewy body dementia.

These case studies illustrate the progression of different types of dementia. But remember, every individual's experience with dementia is unique. The progression can be influenced by many factors, including the specific type of dementia, the person's overall health, and their care environment.

How Different Stages Affect Patients and Caregivers

"Caregiving often calls us to lean into love we didn't know possible." - Tia Walker.

Alzheimer's and dementia are not easy to deal with. The stages can seem like a storm for those in the midst of it. But, just like a storm, they pass. Each stage brings trials for the patient and you, the caregiver. Yet, each stage also brings its own form of growth and understanding.

In the early stages of Alzheimer's and dementia, the changes are subtle. Your loved one may forget familiar names or misplace items. At times, they may seem just fine. But then, they may not recall a recent conversation. This stage can be confusing for both of you. It's like standing at the sea's edge, unsure of what's to come.

As the caregiver, you may feel a range of emotions. Fear, confusion, and frustration are common. Yet, this stage also allows for planning. It's time to discuss care wishes and legal matters. It's also time to seek support from others who have been there.

The middle stages of Alzheimer's and dementia bring more noticeable changes. Memory loss becomes more evident. Your loved one may get lost in familiar places. They may have trouble with daily tasks. Their personality may change. This stage can be like navigating through choppy waters.

Caregiving in this stage can become more demanding. You may need to assist with daily tasks. You may have to manage problematic behaviors. Yet, you also have the chance to connect in new ways. Music, art, or photos can spark memories and create moments of joy.

When Alzheimer's and dementia progress to the late stages, the changes are profound. Your loved one may lose their ability to communicate. They may not recognize you. They may need help with all daily tasks. This stage can feel like being in the eye of the storm, where all is calm, and yet all is not.

Caregiving in this stage requires a deep well of patience and love. You may need to provide round-the-clock care. Or, you may need to make decisions about nursing homes or hospice care. Yet, amidst the challenges, there is also the chance to simply be with your loved one, to hold their hand, to offer comfort through your presence.

The stages of Alzheimer's and dementia are not linear. They can wax and wane. They can overlap. And they can differ from person to person. Understanding these stages can help you as a caregiver. It can help you prepare. It can help you adapt. And it can help you find the strength to weather the storm.

Each stage of Alzheimer's and dementia affects both the patient and caregiver in unique ways. These stages can be challenging, but they can also offer opportunities for growth, connection, and love. The key is to remember that you are not alone. There is help and support available. And, above all, there is always hope.

Through it all, remember that your role as a caregiver is not just about providing care. It's also about showing love, respect, and dignity to your loved one. It's about finding ways to connect, even when words fail. And it's about finding strength within yourself, even when the storm seems unending.

While Alzheimer's and dementia can change many things, they cannot take away the love between you and your loved one. That love remains through every stage, every storm, and every calm. It's the love that will guide you, sustain you, and ultimately empower you.

Chapter Two
Diagnosis and Treatment Options

Seeking a Diagnosis

"An accurate diagnosis is the first step towards effective treatment. It's the key to understanding the problem and finding the best way to manage it." - Anonymous.

When you notice changes in your loved one's behavior or memory, it can be a worrying time. The first step in managing this change is seeking a diagnosis. This process might seem daunting, but it is crucial. It forms the foundation for the care and support that follow.

It involves several medical tests and evaluations. These are not just to confirm the presence of the disease. They also help rule out other possible causes of the symptoms. These can include vitamin deficiencies, thyroid problems, or depression.

Doctors will usually begin with a physical exam. This helps them understand the overall health of the patient. They will also look for any signs of other conditions that could be causing memory problems and conduct a neurological exam. This exam tests for problems with balance, sensory function, and other signs of brain disorders. It can help pinpoint the cause of the symptoms.

Medical professionals will also use cognitive and neuropsychological tests. These assessments measure memory, problem-solving skills, attention span, counting skills, and language abilities. The results give a clear picture of the patient's mental function.

The doctors may also request brain imaging. An MRI or a CT scan can show brain size and shape. It can also identify any noticeable abnormalities. These images can help doctors see if the symptoms are due to Alzheimer's or another brain disorder.

Lab tests can also be a part of the diagnostic process. These tests can check for conditions that can affect memory or cognition. They might include checking vitamin B12 levels or thyroid function tests.

Although the process of seeking a diagnosis for Alzheimer's or dementia can be long and complex, it is a vital step in ensuring your loved one receives the right care. Remember, an early diagnosis can make a significant difference.

It is also important to seek out the right professionals. Quite often family members use the professionals that are comfortable to them, resulting in a misdiagnosis. Search for medical professionals that specialize in cognitive disorders. A wrong diagnosis can delay proper treatment.

Once the diagnosis is confirmed, the focus shifts to the treatment options.

The treatment not only aims to manage the symptoms, it also works towards maintaining mental function, managing behavioral symptoms, and slowing down the disease's progression.

The treatment plan for Alzheimer's or dementia is often multi-faceted. It includes medication, non-drug therapies, and lifestyle changes.

Real-Life Accounts of Diagnosis Experiences

"The first step toward change is awareness." - Nathaniel Branden.

Living with Alzheimer's and dementia is a life-altering experience. It is a journey that begins with a diagnosis. It's a moment that's hard to forget. The doctor's words may have seemed like a blur, but the feeling remains. It's a mix of shock, confusion, and fear. The doctor's words echo in your mind. Alzheimer's. Dementia. These illnesses are real, and they've entered your life.

For many people, the first signs of Alzheimer's or dementia are subtle. They might forget a name, lose track of time, or misplace familiar objects. For some, the changes are so gradual that they barely notice them. But for others, the warning signs are more pronounced. They might become lost in familiar places, struggle with everyday tasks, or start acting out of character. In any case, these early signs are often the first clue that something is not right.

When the diagnosis comes, it can feel like a punch in the gut. It's a moment that turns your world upside down. You may feel a rush of emotions - fear, anger, sadness, denial. You question why this is happening and what the future holds. The uncertainty can be overwhelming. But amidst the chaos, there is a glimmer of hope. This diagnosis is not the end. It's a new beginning. It's a chance to learn, adapt, and find new ways to live and love beyond memory loss.

Accepting the diagnosis is the first step on this journey. It's a hard pill to swallow, but it's necessary. Understanding what Alzheimer's and dementia are, and what they mean for your loved one, is crucial. It paves the way for effective treatment and care strategies. It allows you to prepare for the challenges ahead and find ways to improve your loved one's quality of life. Education is a powerful tool in this battle. It's important to learn as much as you can about these conditions. The more you know, the better equipped you'll be to support your loved one. There are many resources available, from books and online articles to support groups and health professionals. Make use of these resources. Lean on them for guidance and support.

Your loved one's journey with Alzheimer's or dementia is unique. Their symptoms, progression, and response to treatment will vary. It's important to work closely with their healthcare team to tailor a care plan that fits their needs. Regular check-ups and open communication with their doctors are key.

The Emotional Impact of Receiving a Diagnosis

"The greatest discovery of my generation is that a human being can alter his life by altering his attitudes." - William James.

When we first hear of a loved one's diagnosis, shock is the first emotion. It hits hard. The world seems to stop. "Alzheimer's" or "dementia" are words that carry a lot of weight. They change things. They can make us feel as if life, as we know it, is about to end. But, it is vital to know that a diagnosis is not the end. It's a new phase in life, one we can face with courage and grace.

Fear often follows shock. The unknown is scary. We tend to fear what we can't control. And dementia or Alzheimer's? They are diseases we can't control. But remember, fear is a natural reaction. It's okay to feel scared. It's important to accept this fear, to let it be a part of the process.
After fear, comes grief. We grieve for the person we knew. We grieve for the future we imagined. Grief, like fear, is a natural response. It's a part of the process. It's a sign of love. It's a sign that you care. And it's through this grief that we can find strength. Strength to face the days ahead. Strength to care for our loved one.

As we grapple with grief, we may feel anger. Why us? Why our loved one? Anger is a common response when life doesn't go as planned. It's okay to feel angry. It's okay to ask why. But let's not let anger consume us. Let's use it as a catalyst. A catalyst for change. A catalyst for action.

In the midst of all these emotions, there may be a sense of relief. Yes, relief. A diagnosis can provide answers. Answers to questions we've had for a while. It can explain changes in behavior or memory. It can provide a sense of closure, even if it's not the closure we wanted.

Remember, there is no 'right' way to react to a diagnosis. Every person is unique. Every journey is different. You may feel all these emotions. Or, you may feel none of them. You may feel them in a different order.

Or, you may feel them all at once. It's okay. Your feelings are valid. Your reactions are valid.

As time moves on, you may find acceptance. Acceptance of the diagnosis. Acceptance of the new reality. This acceptance doesn't mean you're happy about the situation. It means you're ready to face it. You're ready to take on the challenge. You're ready to love and care for your loved one, no matter what.

Medical Interventions

"The art of medicine consists of amusing the patient while nature cures the disease." - Voltaire.

In the fight against Alzheimer's and dementia, medical science is our ally. It offers us a range of treatments. These treatments won't cure the disease. But they can help in managing symptoms. They can slow down the disease's progress. They can improve the quality of life for patients. And they can ease the burden on caregivers.

Medications are the first line of defense. These are drugs that can help with memory loss, sleep problems, and mood changes. The drugs can also help manage other symptoms of Alzheimer's and dementia. These include confusion, hallucinations, and agitation.

Donepezil is a common drug used in Alzheimer's treatment. It belongs to a class of drugs known as cholinesterase inhibitors. These drugs work by boosting levels of a chemical messenger involved in memory and judgment. Donepezil may also help with some behavioral symptoms.

Another drug used is memantine. It works in a different way. It regulates the activity of glutamate. Glutamate is another chemical messenger. It's involved in learning and memory. Memantine can help slow the progression of symptoms in moderate to severe Alzheimer's disease.
A newer class of drugs is the BACE inhibitors. These drugs aim to change the disease process itself. They try to block an enzyme involved in the production of abnormal amyloid protein. This protein forms plaques in the brain of Alzheimer's patients.

Apart from drugs, there are also non-drug treatments. These include physical activity, healthy diet, and mental stimulation. These can help slow cognitive decline in Alzheimer's patients. Some studies suggest that regular physical activity and a diet rich in fruits, vegetables and whole grains can help protect brain health.

Cognitive stimulation is another important strategy. This can involve activities such as reading, puzzles, and playing musical instruments. These activities keep the mind active and engaged. They help slow the progression of Alzheimer's and dementia.

Behavioral interventions are also useful. These include techniques to manage behavior. They can help with common issues such as aggression, agitation, and sleep disturbances. Examples include distraction, redirection, and the use of simple, clear language.

Counseling and support groups can provide emotional support. They can help both caregivers and patients cope with the disease. These resources can help caregivers understand the disease. They can make them feel less alone. They can provide tips and strategies for managing challenging behaviors.

The Latest Advancements

"The future is already here, it's just not evenly distributed." - William Gibson.

The world of medical science is always evolving. New findings come to light, paving the way for better treatments and hope for those grappling with diseases like Alzheimer's and dementia. As caregivers, staying informed about these advancements is key. It equips you with the knowledge to better care for your loved ones and understand the complexities of their condition.

In recent years, several medical professionals have shared their insights on the latest advancements in Alzheimer's and dementia treatment. These insights are crucial for caregivers, as they offer a glimpse into the future of these conditions. They provide hope and show that the medical community is working tirelessly to find more effective treatments and, ultimately, a cure.

One such advancement is the development of new drugs that slow down the progression of Alzheimer's. While a cure is not yet available, these drugs offer hope. They can delay the onset of severe symptoms, allowing patients to maintain their independence for longer. These medications work by targeting the underlying causes of Alzheimer's, such as the build-up of plaques in the brain.

Another promising area of research is the role of lifestyle changes in preventing or slowing down dementia. Studies have shown that regular physical activity, a healthy diet, and mental stimulation can all play a part in keeping the brain healthy. As a caregiver, you can incorporate these elements into the daily routine of your loved one, helping to bolster their cognitive health.

The use of technology in Alzheimer's and dementia care is also gaining traction. From memory-aiding apps to GPS devices that prevent wandering, tech advancements are proving to be valuable tools for caregivers. These tools can offer a sense of security and make day-to-day caregiving tasks more manageable.

Genetic research is another burgeoning field in the fight against Alzheimer's and dementia. Scientists are working to identify the genes responsible for these conditions. This research could lead to early detection and personalized treatment plans, tailored to the genetic makeup of each individual.

The insights from these medical professionals are not just about the future of Alzheimer's and dementia treatment. They also offer practical strategies that you can implement right now. Whether it's incorporating more physical activity into your loved one's routine or exploring the use of technology in care, these advancements provide actionable ways to improve the caregiving experience.

It's important to remember that while these advancements offer hope, every individual's experience with Alzheimer's and dementia is unique. What works for one person may not work for another. Patience, compassion, and a willingness to adapt are essential qualities for any caregiver.

Managing Expectations Regarding Treatment Outcomes

"The greatest healing therapy is friendship and love," said Hubert H. Humphrey, a sentiment that is very true in our discussion today.

When dealing with Alzheimer's and dementia, it's vital to grasp the role of treatment. It's not about a cure, as, sadly, we don't have one yet. It's about managing symptoms. It's about making life better for your loved one and for you, the caregiver.

Let's start with a basic fact. Alzheimer's and dementia are progressive conditions. Over time, memory loss gets worse. It's a hard truth, but knowing this can help you set sensible expectations.

The goal of treatment is to manage the progression of the disease, enhance the quality of life, and extend independence. Medications play a crucial role in achieving these goals by alleviating symptoms such as memory loss and confusion. Some can help with slowing down the disease. But they can't stop the disease. New treatments are on the horizon everyday. The hope is that some day, there will be a cure.

Not every drug works the same way for every person. What's more, the effect of drugs may lessen over time. It's key to discuss this with your loved one's doctor. They can explain what to expect from each medicine.

A crucial part of treatment is non-drug care. This might mean changes to the home. It could also mean daily routines that bring comfort. It's about making life simpler and less confusing for your loved one.

Non-drug care can also include activities. Music, art, or walks in nature can bring joy. They can help your loved one feel calm and connected. As a caregiver, it's a good idea to explore these options.

Also, take note of diet and exercise. A healthy body can often mean a healthier mind. Regular movement and good food can help manage symptoms.

Sleep is another key factor. Many people with Alzheimer's have trouble sleeping. This can make symptoms worse. So, good sleep routines can be a part of care.

Alternative and Complementary Approaches

"Natural forces within us are the true healers of disease." - Hippocrates.

When we think of Alzheimer's and dementia, we often focus on the medical side of treatment. But there is more that we can explore. We can look at other ways to support our loved ones. There are different ways to help that don't involve pills or doctors. They are called alternative and complementary approaches. These are ways to care for the whole person, not just the disease.

Holistic approaches are about treating the whole person. They focus on the mind, body, and spirit. This is different from traditional medicine, which often just looks at the physical symptoms of a disease. Some examples of holistic therapies include yoga, meditation, and art therapy. These therapies aim to reduce stress and improve the quality of life.

Yoga, for example, is a gentle form of exercise that can be adapted for people with Alzheimer's and dementia. It can help improve balance and flexibility, which can reduce the risk of falls. But it can also help reduce stress and promote a feeling of calm. This can be beneficial for both the person with dementia and the caregiver.

Meditation is another holistic therapy that can be useful. It can help to calm the mind and reduce stress. It can also improve focus and attention, which can be beneficial for people with dementia. There are different types of meditation, including mindfulness meditation and loving-kindness meditation. These can be done alone or in a group setting, and there are many resources available to help you get started.

Art therapy can also be beneficial. It provides a way for people with dementia to express themselves. It can also help to improve mood and reduce stress. Art therapy can involve drawing, painting, or even sculpting. It can be a fun and relaxing activity that can be done together.

Along with holistic therapies, there are also non-pharmaceutical therapies to consider. These include things like music therapy, aromatherapy, and pet therapy. These therapies can help to improve mood and reduce agitation. They can also provide a sense of comfort and familiarity.

Music therapy, for example, can be very effective. Music can help to calm and soothe. It can also trigger memories and emotions. This can be especially beneficial for people with Alzheimer's and dementia, as music can often reach parts of the brain that other forms of communication cannot.

Aromatherapy involves the use of essential oils to promote well-being. Some research suggests that certain scents, like lavender and rosemary, may help to improve memory and cognition in people with dementia. However, it's important to use these oils safely and to talk to a healthcare provider before starting any new therapy.

Pet therapy can also be beneficial. Animals can provide companionship and comfort. They can also help to reduce stress and anxiety. Some studies have shown that spending time with animals can improve mood and behavior in people with dementia.

Finding Success with Alternative Approaches

"The only way to do great work is to love what you do." - Steve Jobs.

Alzheimer's and dementia can be a tough journey. But, you are not alone. Many families have walked this path. They have used different approaches and found success. This section is about their stories. It is about their trials, their errors, and their triumphs. It aims to give you hope and new ideas.

One family found music therapy to be very effective. Ellie's mom had severe dementia. She was often confused and upset. But, when Ellie played her mom's favorite songs, the change was clear. Her mom calmed down. She even hummed along to some of the tunes. It was a breakthrough for Ellie. She saw that music could reach her mom when words could not.

Another family discovered the value of routine. John's dad had Alzheimer's. He was often disoriented. But, when John set up a daily routine, his dad responded well. He knew what to expect. The routine gave him a sense of control. It helped to ease his anxiety.

Keeping a positive attitude was a key factor for Sarah's family. Her grandma had dementia. It was tough to see her decline. But, Sarah's family chose to stay positive. They celebrated the good days. They shared laughs and made memories. Their positive outlook helped them to cope. It also lifted the spirit of their grandma.

Pets can also be a source of comfort and joy. Mike's wife had Alzheimer's. She often felt alone and scared. But, when Mike brought home a small dog, things changed. His wife bonded with the dog. She found comfort in his company. The dog was a source of love and companionship for her.

Diet changes also made a big difference for some families. Emily's mom had dementia. She had lost a lot of weight. Emily decided to try a diet high in healthy fats. She served foods like avocados and nuts. Her mom started to gain weight. Her energy levels also improved.

Then, there is the case of Bob and his dad. His dad had Alzheimer's. He often had trouble sleeping. Bob tried many different things. But, what worked best was a simple change in environment. He made his dad's room darker and quieter. His dad started to sleep better. His mood also improved.

The use of art therapy was a game-changer for Linda's family. Her husband had dementia. He had lost interest in many things. But, art therapy sparked his creativity. He began to paint and draw. It gave him a way to express his feelings. It also gave him a sense of purpose.

These are just a few examples of alternative approaches. They may or may not work for your family. But, they show that there are many ways to provide care. They show that it is possible to find joy and success on this journey.

The Importance of a Holistic Care Plan

"Taking care of someone who once took care of us is the highest honor." - Tia Walker.

The role you play as a caregiver for a loved one with Alzheimer's or dementia is profound. It's a path filled with tests of patience, endurance, and emotional resilience. But remember, it's also an act of immense love and devotion.

To navigate this path effectively, you need a plan. Not just any plan, but a holistic one. A holistic care plan considers the whole person, their physical, emotional, social, and spiritual needs. It's not just about managing symptoms, but also about improving the quality of life for both you and your loved one.

But why is a holistic approach so crucial? Let's start with the basics. Alzheimer's and dementia are not just about memory loss. These conditions affect the entire brain, and by extension, the whole person. Changes in mood, behavior, and physical health are all part of the journey. A holistic care plan takes into account all these changes. It helps you understand how best to support your loved one in all aspects of their life. For instance, a good diet and regular exercise can help manage some physical symptoms. Music or art therapy can be soothing and provide emotional relief. Social activities can keep your loved one engaged and help maintain their sense of self.

Remember, this plan is not just about your loved one. It's also about you. Caregiving is demanding, and it's easy to neglect your own needs. But remember, you can't pour from an empty cup. You need to take care of your own physical and emotional health to be the best caregiver you can be.

Consider your own diet, exercise routine, and need for rest. Seek support from friends, family, or caregiver support groups. Make time for activities you enjoy. This is not selfish but necessary.

Developing a holistic care plan also means having difficult conversations about end-of-life care. While challenging to discuss, it's crucial to respect your loved one's wishes. It also helps you to prepare and make informed decisions when the time comes.

Chapter Three
The Caregiver's Role and Responsibilities

"In the heart of every caregiver is a knowing that we are all connected. As I do for you, I do for me." - Tia Walker.

Becoming a caregiver is not a step most of us plan for, yet it's a role many of us find ourselves in. It's a shift filled with emotions, challenges, and rewards that can truly change our lives. Let's look at some personal stories of individuals who took on this role, caring for loved ones with Alzheimer's and dementia.

Mary was a high school teacher in her late 40s when she took on caregiving for her mother. Her mother had always been the rock of their family. But Alzheimer's changed that. Mary had to step in to help her navigate her day-to-day life. It was hard, but it brought them closer. They found joy in shared moments, even as they faced the challenges Alzheimer's brought.

John was a retired police officer who became a full-time caregiver for his wife. She had always been his life partner, and now he had to take on a new role. It was a difficult transition, but he found purpose in caring for her. He learned about patience, compassion, and the strength of their bond.

Sue was a young woman in her 30s when her father was diagnosed with dementia. She had a full-time job and a young family of her own. But she stepped up, sharing care duties with her siblings and adjusting her life to accommodate her father's needs. It was a challenge, but she found strength in her family and their love for their father.

These stories are unique, yet they share common threads. Each person had to step into the role of caregiver, facing both the challenges and rewards it brought. Each person had to learn about Alzheimer's and dementia, understand their loved one's needs, and find ways to support them.

Becoming a caregiver is a journey filled with many emotions. It can be challenging but also a role that can bring great rewards. It's a role that requires patience, compassion, and understanding. It's a role that can deepen our connections with our loved ones, even as we navigate the challenges of Alzheimer's and dementia.

As a caregiver, you play a crucial role in your loved one's life. You provide support, care, and love. You're there to help them navigate their day-to-day lives, helping them maintain their dignity and quality of life. And while it's a challenging role, it's also one that can bring great rewards.

In your role as a caregiver, you become an advocate for your loved one. You're their voice when they can't speak for themselves, their support when they feel lost. You're their source of comfort and their beacon of hope. It's a role that demands a lot from you, but it's also one that can bring great fulfillment.

Caregiving can also bring about personal growth. It can help you develop skills and traits that can benefit you in other areas of your life. Skills like patience, compassion, resilience, and problem-solving can all be strengthened through your role as a caregiver.

While caregiving for someone with Alzheimer's or dementia can be challenging, it can also bring moments of joy. When you connect with your loved one and share a laugh or a memory, moments can bring light into the most challenging days. Even as you navigate the difficulties, holding onto these moments of joy is essential.

Emotional Challenges and Adjustments Required

"The emotion that can break your heart is sometimes the very one that heals it."
- Nicholas Sparks.

Living with Alzheimer's or dementia in your household can be a roller coaster of emotions. You may feel love, joy, and happiness at times. But you may also feel sadness, anger, and frustration. As a caregiver, it's crucial to understand these emotions and learn how to manage them.

One of the first emotions you may feel is denial. It's common to think that the signs of Alzheimer's or dementia are just normal aging. You may brush off the symptoms or make excuses for their behavior. It is also important to note that other friends and family members who don't see the loved one regularly, may notice these changes before you do. It's easy to deny there's a problem when the changes seem subtle. But denial can prevent you from getting the help your loved one needs. It's important to recognize this emotion and seek medical advice if you suspect Alzheimer's or dementia.

Fear is another emotion you may have. You may worry about what the future holds or how you'll manage as your loved one's condition worsens. To cope with fear, focus on the present. Take one day at a time and make the most of the good moments.

Guilt is a common emotion, too. You may feel guilty for not doing enough or for feeling frustrated or angry. Remember, it's normal to feel this way. You're doing the best you can. Take time to care for yourself and seek support if you need it.

Anger can surface when you feel overwhelmed or frustrated. You may feel angry at your loved one, at the situation, or even at yourself. It's okay to feel angry. But it's important to express your anger in healthy ways. Find outlets for your anger, like exercise or talking to a friend.

Sadness and grief can come as you witness your loved one's decline. You may feel a sense of loss for the person your loved one used to be. These feelings are normal. It's important to allow yourself to grieve. Seek support from others who understand what you're going through.

Finally, you may feel isolated or alone. Caregiving can be a lonely task. You may feel like no one understands what you're going through. But you're not alone. Reach out to support groups or other caregivers. They can offer comfort and understanding.

As a caregiver, you'll also need to make adjustments in your life. You may need to change your routine or take on new roles. You may need to learn new skills or seek help from others. These changes can be challenging. But with patience and flexibility, you can adapt.

One of the biggest adjustments is accepting your new role as a caregiver. This role can bring new responsibilities and challenges. But it can also be rewarding. You can make a difference in your loved one's life.

Another adjustment is learning to balance caregiving with other parts of your life. You may need to juggle work, family, and personal time. It's crucial to find a balance that works for you. Remember, taking care of yourself is just as important as caring for your loved one.

Also, you'll need to learn to communicate effectively with your loved one. Alzheimer's and dementia can affect communication skills. You'll need to be patient and understanding. Use simple, clear sentences and give your loved one time to respond.

The Importance of Self-Care for Caregivers

"Self-care is never a selfish act—it is simply good stewardship of the only gift I have, the gift I was put on earth to offer to others." - Parker Palmer.

Caregiving is a noble act. It's a task that calls for deep empathy, patience, and love. Yet, it can also be strenuous and draining. When you're caring for a loved one with Alzheimer's or dementia, the task can become even more challenging. Hence, it's paramount to remember the importance of self-care in this role.

Taking care of yourself isn't a luxury. It's a need. It's the fuel that keeps you going, even in tough times. When you're re-fueled, you can offer the best care to your loved one. You're more patient. You're more understanding. And you're more present.

Being present is crucial in caregiving. Yet, it's hard to be present when you're exhausted or stressed. That's where self-care comes in. It helps you manage your stress. It helps you recharge. And it helps you stay healthy.

When we speak of self-care, we mean more than just physical health. Yes, eating well, getting enough sleep, and regular exercise are essential. But self-care also involves your mental and emotional health. It consists of taking time for yourself, doing things that bring you joy, and seeking support when needed.

Life with a loved one who has Alzheimer's or dementia can be unpredictable. There will be good days and challenging days. In the midst of it all, you need to find balance. You need to find time for yourself. And you need to take care of your needs.

Caring for your needs doesn't mean you're neglecting your loved one. In fact, by taking care of yourself, you're better equipped to care for them. You're more patient. You're more empathetic. And you're more resilient.

You may feel guilty at first. You may feel like you're being selfish. But remember, self-care isn't selfish. It's essential. It's the act of giving yourself permission to replenish your energy.

Self-care isn't a one-time act. It's a continuous process. It's a habit that needs to be cultivated. And it's a mindset that needs to be embraced. Remember, you matter, your well-being matters. And taking care of yourself is part of your caregiving journey.

In the face of Alzheimer's or dementia, you're not just a caregiver. You're a lifeline. You're a source of comfort and love. And you're a source of strength. But to be that lifeline, you need to care for yourself. You need to keep your light shining bright.

Practical Caregiving Techniques

"The care you give to yourself is the care you give to your loved one," said former caregiver, Dana Tyson.

Providing care for someone with Alzheimer's or dementia is a task that demands both love and skill. It is a journey filled with unique hurdles but also with moments of deep connection and profound understanding. In this section, we will go through some practical tips and techniques to help you in your daily caregiving tasks.

Effective communication is a cornerstone of caregiving. When interacting with a loved one who has Alzheimer's or dementia, try to keep your language simple and concise. Avoid complex sentences and big words that might confuse them. Try to explain things in simple terms instead of lecturing. Lecturing can cause stress, hurt, confusion and frustration for the person with Alzheimer's. Avoid sentences like, "I told you that yesterday" or "Why don't you listen to me." Be patient, giving them time to process what you've said and respond.

Another critical aspect of caregiving is creating a safe and familiar environment. Your loved one may feel disoriented or anxious due to their memory loss. Maintaining a stable daily routine and organized living space can help alleviate some of these feelings.

It's important to stimulate their mind and body. Simple activities such as puzzles, games, and walks can keep them active and engaged. These activities can also strengthen your bond with your loved one, providing shared moments of joy and achievement.

Nutrition and hydration are crucial. Alzheimer's and dementia can sometimes cause a decrease in appetite or forgetfulness about eating. Regular, nutritious meals and plenty of water are vital for their health. Be patient during meal times, and encourage them to eat and drink.

Personal grooming can be a challenging task for those with Alzheimer's or dementia. Assist them with tasks like brushing their teeth, bathing, and dressing. Make these activities as stress-free as possible, providing reassurance and gentle guidance.

Remember, it's okay to ask for help. If you're feeling overwhelmed, seek support from friends, family, or professional caregivers. There are also numerous support groups and resources available for caregivers of those with Alzheimer's or dementia.

While providing care, remember to take care of yourself too. Your well-being is equally important. Try to maintain a balanced diet, exercise regularly, and take some time each day for relaxation and self-care.

Managing behavioral changes can be challenging. Your loved one may exhibit changes in mood, agitation, or aggression. In these instances, try to remain calm and patient. Distraction can often help, shifting their attention to a more pleasant topic or activity.

In terms of medical care, ensure that your loved one receives regular check-ups and takes their prescribed medication. It's also worth discussing with their healthcare provider about any alternative or complementary therapies that might be beneficial.

Tips for Maintaining Patience and Empathy

"Patience is not the ability to wait, but the ability to keep a good attitude while waiting." - Joyce Meyer.

Being a caregiver to someone with Alzheimer's or dementia is no easy task. The task can be draining, both physically and emotionally. It is a role that demands both patience and empathy. Here, we share practical tips to help you maintain these two vital qualities.

First, try to keep in mind that the person you're caring for is not at fault. It's the disease that's causing the changes in their behavior. This thought can help you stay patient when things get tough. It's also crucial to remember that everyone makes mistakes. It's not their fault when your loved one forgets something or behaves oddly. It's just the nature of the disease.

Secondly, it's essential to take care of yourself. You can't pour from an empty cup. Ensure you get enough rest, eat healthily, and take time for yourself. This self-care will help you stay patient and empathetic towards your loved one. When you feel good, you're more likely to have the energy to provide the care your loved one needs.

Thirdly, try to put yourself in their shoes. Imagine what it's like to forget the faces of loved ones or struggle with everyday tasks. This exercise can help you cultivate empathy for the person you're caring for. It can also help you understand their feelings and actions better.

Also, learn as much as you can about Alzheimer's and dementia. Understanding these conditions can help you manage your expectations. It can also help you communicate more effectively with your loved one. The more you know, the better you'll be able to provide the care they need.

Next, try to stay positive. It's easy to get overwhelmed by the challenges of caregiving. But try to focus on the good moments. Celebrate small victories, like a successful day of activities or a calm evening. These moments of joy can help you stay patient and empathetic.

In addition, it's important to seek support. Join a support group, talk to friends, or seek professional help if needed. Sharing your experiences and hearing others' stories can help you cope. It can also provide practical tips and a sense of community.

Navigating Legal and Financial Aspects

"Legal matters are the anchors of life's ship, not the sails. But they help keep the ship steady in the storm." - Anonymous.

In dealing with Alzheimer's and dementia, we often get so caught up in day-to-day care that we overlook the legal and financial aspects. These elements are crucial to ensure the well-being of your loved one and yourself. In this section, we will discuss two main areas - power of attorney and advance directives.

A power of attorney is a legal document that allows you to appoint someone to act on your loved one's behalf. This person, known as the agent, can make decisions about finances and health care when your loved one is unable to do so. It's essential to establish a power of attorney as early as possible while your loved one can still understand and consent to the arrangement. Neglecting this crucial legal aspect could lead to significant anxiety and substantial legal costs in the future.

Choosing the right person as the agent is vital. This person should be trustworthy, reliable, and capable of making difficult decisions. Choosing someone familiar with your loved one's situation and wishes is often a good idea. Remember, the agent's role is to act in the best interest of your loved one.

On the other hand, an advance directive is a legal document that outlines your loved one's wishes regarding future medical care. It comes into play when they can no longer communicate or make decisions. This document can help ensure that your loved one's healthcare preferences are respected, even when they cannot express them themselves.

There are two primary forms of advance directives: living wills and medical power of attorney. A living will states your loved one's wishes for end-of-life care. It may specify whether they want life-sustaining treatments, such as resuscitation or artificial feeding.

A medical power of attorney, also known as a healthcare proxy, appoints a person to make medical decisions on your loved one's behalf. This person should know your loved one's values and wishes about their health care. They will have the authority to make medical decisions when your loved one can't.

Both these documents should be discussed in-depth with your loved one while they still have the cognitive ability to express their wishes. It might be difficult to broach such sensitive topics, but it's essential for their well-being and peace of mind.

Keep in mind that laws regarding power of attorney and advance directives can vary from state to state. It's a good idea to consult with a legal professional who specializes in elder law. They can guide you through the process and ensure all documents are correctly prepared according to your state's laws.

These legal tools are not only about preparing for the worst. They are about ensuring that your loved one's wishes are respected, and they receive the care they desire. They can also provide guidance and direction as you navigate the complexities of caregiving and ensure that you are making decisions that align with your loved one's preferences.

Financial Planning and Resources for Long-Term Care

"Failing to plan is planning to fail." This quote by Benjamin Franklin is still

true today, especially when dealing with long-term care for a loved one with Alzheimer's or dementia.

Financial planning is a critical step in preparing for the long haul. It's not just about the money. It's about peace of mind. Knowing you have a plan can reduce stress. It can free you up to focus on care and love. Think about the costs. Care for Alzheimer's or dementia can be pricey. Costs could include in-home care, adult daycare, or a memory care facility. You also have to factor in medical costs. These can consist of doctors, medicine, and therapy.

Start by seeking out a financial advisor. They can help map out a plan. This plan could include savings, investments, and insurance. Financial advisors can also help you understand tax breaks for caregivers.

Long-term care insurance is another option to consider. This type of insurance helps cover the cost of care not covered by health insurance. Long-term insurance can also help pay for in-home care or memory care facilities.

There are also public programs that can help. Medicare and Medicaid can provide assistance. Veterans' benefits may also be an option. Each program has its own rules and eligibility.

Another resource to tap into is the Alzheimer's Association. This group offers a wealth of information. They can guide you to financial and legal resources. They also provide support groups and training for caregivers.

Remember your own financial health. As a caregiver, you may face your own financial strain. You might have to reduce work hours or even quit your job. Make sure to factor this into your plan. Look for ways to reduce costs. There might be ways to save on care or medical costs. For example, some drug companies offer discounts on prescriptions.

Dementia Care Checklist

Your loved one's diagnosis of Alzheimer's disease or other dementia has likely thrown your family life into a bit of chaos. Thankfully, the senior care industry has rallied around those with Alzheimer's disease and other dementias over the past few decades.

You are now able to access dementia care communities that are carefully designed with the senior in mind. However, finding the perfect dementia care unit or community can still be a daunting task. In order to make the best decision about dementia care possible, it is good to visit at least three communities more than once.

Using your loved one's challenges and prognosis as a lens, you can make the best decision that suits your current situation. By separating out the "good enough" communities from the "best of the best" communities, you can get a good start on your quest to find a dementia care community.

However, you probably still have a few choices to make. Here is an easy checklist to help you be sure that you are asking the right questions and looking for the right things that can make your decision a bit easier.

Some of these questions are posed to you, while others are written so that you know the wording to use to ask the dementia care community professional.

Remember: You can follow up with communities as much as you want via phone calls, requested tours, or other events. Gather all the information you need in order to make a well-informed decision that you will feel good about.

Once you have decided on possible facilities, it is also a good idea to have your loved one on several wait lists as many memory care centers can fill up quickly and availability is unpredictable.

Another important consideration is to consider in advance what items will be taken to the memory care center. Nothing of any real value should be taken and all items should be labeled. Things may disappear. But if properly marked, they eventually make their way back.

Ask your loved one what personal things they'd like to bring with them-radio or music device, TV with DVD player and DVDs of their favorite programs or movies, photos and artwork. Ask early on what they like. Photos are wonderful, but photos that include them with family members at a place that has fond memories seem to have more value. Artwork that means something to them, even it is just the bright colors, seems to be most important, especially when they just need something to focus on.

ENVIRONMENT AND LOCATION
  • Is the location convenient for me and other family members to visit

frequently?

- Is the parking situation for visitors welcoming and easy to navigate?
- Is the community located in a quiet, residential neighborhood?
- If the community is in a city, will the noises be distracting or concerning to my loved one?
- Is the community in a city or location that my loved one will enjoy?
- Is the community located near places I can take my loved one to on my own during visits, such as restaurants or shopping?
- Does the community smell and look clean?
- Are there flowers and plants inside and outside of the community?
- Are there animals in the community (fish, birds, a community dog, etc.), and how will that affect my loved one?
- May I bring my dog to visit, if my loved one would like that?
- Are there places that I may visit with my loved one besides his or her room or apartment?
- Is there a place available for a larger family gathering within the community that we may rent or reserve if needed?
- Does the community seem lively but not chaotic?
- Do the residents seem happy and engaged?
- Do the residents seem well-groomed? Is there an outdoor space that residents can easily access and enjoy?

APARTMENT AND AMENITIES

- Are there private apartments available?
- Do the apartments come furnished with certain items?
- What are we allowed to bring in from home?
- Who is in charge of hanging up pictures, shelves, etc.?
- Will someone be available to help us move in?

- Are there cueing devices (such as photos or shadow boxes) outside apartments to let residents know which one is theirs?
- What safety precautions are in the bathroom?
- Are residents allowed to choose when they take a shower?
- Is there a place for a resident to take a bath, should he or she want to?
- Is there a call-light system?
- Where is the nursing station in regard to the apartments?
- How often does housekeeping visit my loved one's apartment?
- Do you do laundry here, or am I responsible for doing it?
- If you do laundry here, do I need to take any steps in order to prepare the clothing (e.g., labeling)?
- If my loved one is nervous about a housekeeper coming into his or her apartment to clean, what can you do to make that less stressful for my loved one while still ensuring that the apartment is clean?

MEDICAL MANAGEMENT

- Do you have a relationship with my loved one's doctor?
- Are there specialists (podiatrists, dentists, etc.) who visit the unit regularly?
- Will you work with the pharmacy to order new medications and refill old ones, or do I need to do that?
- Can you support my loved one's chronic condition with _______________ (oxygen use, etc.)?
- May my loved one have a walker in this unit? A wheelchair? An electric scooter?
- How do you inform me and the doctor about any change in my loved one's condition? A fall? An emergency room visit?
- Does my loved one have access to therapy (physical, occupational,

speech) services right here in the unit?

- Does my loved one have access to range-of-motion exercises here in the unit?

STAFFING

- What types of training does your staff receive on an ongoing basis?
- Can you give me a few topics that your staff has been educated about in the past few months?
- Are all staff required to attend training, or is it just the nursing staff?
- Are nurses on staff 24 hours a day?
- Are those nurses RNs or LPNs? Are your caregivers also CNAs?
- What are your staffing ratios for different times of the day?
- Do those fluctuate based on resident needs?
- Do you have volunteers who work with residents, too?

FINANCIAL CONSIDERATIONS

- What is the monthly rent?
- What does this monthly fee include?
- Are there additional costs assessed for more care or assistance? What are those?
- Will you let me know before any prices increase?
- How are prescriptions billed?
- How are other medical services (therapy, dentist visits, etc.) billed?
- Do you accept Medicaid?
- Do you accept my loved one's long-term care or secondary insurance?
- What happens when my loved one can no longer pay for services or rent?
- How much do incontinence products cost? May I bring products in

that I purchase?

- What types of items do I need to purchase and bring (shampoo, razors, etc.)?
- Am I billed for items such as gloves, wipes, or other medical supplies?

ACTIVITIES

- May I meet your activities director and staff?
- May I attend an activity with my loved one?
- Do residents seem engaged and happy when you visit the unit?
- Are there activities on the activity calendar that my loved one would enjoy?
- Are there trips planned on a monthly basis?
- Are there activities planned seven days a week?
- Are there activities planned for the evening times?
- Does the community offer religious services or support that meet my loved one's needs?
- Does the community invite kids into the community for intergenerational programming?
- Does the community offer therapy dog visits to interested residents?
- Are there activities available that encourage exercise and range of motion (sit and be fit, yoga, tai chi, etc.)?
- Are there activities that encourage failure-free conversation (reminiscence groups, etc.)?
- Residents with middle- and late-stage dementia often respond well to multisensory experiences. Does the community offer those (hand massages, sensory stimulation groups, etc.)?
- Are families able to participate in activities with loved ones?
- How do you encourage residents to attend groups?

- If residents are unable to sit for long activities, how do you meet their needs for socialization?
- May residents suggest activities for the community?

DINING

- Is the dining room homelike and welcoming?
- May I observe a meal?
- Does the menu offer choices for residents?
- If residents cannot or do not speak, how do you determine which entree or choice they would like?
- My loved one doesn't like _______________. What options do you have for him or her?
- My loved one cannot use a fork. Do you have healthy finger foods that encourage independence?
- Is there assistance in the dining room during meals?
- Are your chefs experienced in cooking medically recommended diets?
- May residents assist with homelike tasks like setting the table?

FAMILY INVOLVEMENT

- Are families involved in the life of the community?
- Do the visiting hours suit your personal and professional schedule? Do you feel welcome when you enter the building?
- During your tour, do you notice family members or friends visiting?
- Are there educational lectures available for families or friends?
- Are there regularly scheduled Family Nights or other events that encourage participation?
- How are family members notified of upcoming care plans?
- If you live far away or are on vacation, how can the community keep

you updated on the daily life of your loved one?
- Is there a community Facebook, Instagram, or blog page?
- Is there a family newsletter available each month?
- Do the executive director and other management staff make an effort to get to know family members?

UNIQUE CHALLENGES AND CONTINUING CARE
- My loved one has a unique challenge (wandering, aggression, anxiety, etc.). How will you work with that while preserving his or her dignity?
- Is there anything that may jeopardize my loved one's living here?
- When may he or she be asked to move out?
- Will we have ample notice if we are asked to move out?
- Do you work with any skilled nursing communities in the area if my loved one would need inpatient care?

Courtesy of Arbor Terrace of Ashville.
Learn more at https://www.arborcompany.com/locations/northcarolina/asheville.

64

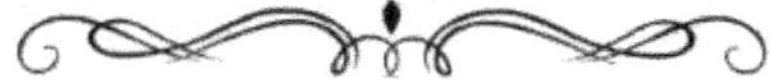

Chapter Four
Communication and Connection

"The best and most beautiful things in the world cannot be seen or even touched - they must be felt with the heart." - Helen Keller.

The power of human connection is beyond measure. It is a bond that unites us, even when words fail. For caregivers dealing with Alzheimer's and dementia, this bond can be a lifeline.

For some caregivers, maintaining connections can be as simple as sharing a favorite song or a cherished family recipe. For others, it may be about taking a walk in a familiar park or looking through family photos. It's about finding those little things that spark joy, ignite memories, and reinforce the bonds of love.

Research supports this approach. Studies show that social interaction can improve the quality of life for people with Alzheimer's and dementia. When caregivers engage with patients on a personal level, it can lead to better emotional well-being for both parties.

But maintaining connections isn't always easy. Alzheimer's can lead to changes in behavior and personality that can be challenging to deal with. Patients may become confused, angry, or withdrawn. In these moments, it's essential to remember the person behind the disease and their life, love, and legacy.

Caregivers like you may wonder how to maintain connections when faced with such obstacles. How do you reach out to someone who seems to be slipping away? The answer lies in love, patience, and understanding.

Strategies for Effective Communication with Your Loved One

"The most important thing in communication is hearing what isn't said." - Peter Drucker.

In the midst of the challenges that come with Alzheimer's and dementia, it's crucial to master the art of effective communication. This doesn't merely mean talking; it's about creating a bridge of understanding. So, how do you go about this?

First, always speak clearly and calmly. Patients with Alzheimer's or dementia may struggle with processing complex sentences. Use simple and direct language, speaking in a gentle and reassuring tone. This will help to prevent confusion and anxiety.

Secondly, maintain eye contact. This non-verbal form of communication can convey empathy, respect, and attentiveness. It's a powerful tool to connect with your loved one on a deeper level, making them feel seen and valued.

Avoid arguing, lecturing or correcting your loved one. It can cause stress, confusion, hurt and frustration. The reality they experience might be different from yours due to memory loss. Instead of attempting to correct them, try to enter their world. This act of empathy can ease tension and foster a better connection.

Patience is key in communicating with a loved one with Alzheimer's or dementia. Allow them ample time to respond during conversations. Rushing them might lead to frustration and stress, hindering effective communication.

Ask simple questions. Ask yes or no questions instead of open-ended questions that may confuse them. This can make it easier for them to respond and participate in the conversation.

Encourage non-verbal communication. If verbal communication becomes difficult, embrace other ways to express feelings and thoughts. This could be through touch, music, art, or even dance. These alternatives can provide comfort and connection.

Be attentive to their body language. A significant part of communication is non-verbal. Paying attention to your loved one's facial expressions, gestures, and body movements can provide valuable insights into their feelings and needs.

Create a calm environment. Loud noises or a chaotic environment can make communication more challenging. A quiet and peaceful setting can enhance focus and understanding during conversations.

Use visual cues and repetition. Visual aids can help in clarifying your points. Also, if necessary, don't hesitate to repeat important information to ensure understanding.

Creative Ways to Engage and Stimulate Memory

"Memory is the diary that we all carry about with us." - Oscar Wilde.

In this battle against Alzheimer's and dementia, let's arm ourselves with the power of memory. Stimulating the brain's capacity to recall can often be an effective way to combat these conditions. Let's look at some creative ways to engage and stimulate memory.

Pictures can serve as a powerful memory stimulant. Create a photo album filled with moments from your loved one's past. Go through it together, allowing them to recall and share stories behind each photo. This practice can bring joy and provide a shared bonding experience.

Music has a unique way of reaching into the memory banks. Create a playlist of your loved one's favorite songs. Listen to them together, and you might find them humming along or even singing. Music can help rekindle old memories and feelings.

Aroma can trigger memories. Certain smells, like the scent of a favorite dish or perfume, can evoke strong memories. Use familiar scents to help your loved one recall events or people from their past.

Engage them in simple household tasks. Folding laundry or setting the table can help stimulate motor functions and recall sequences. These tasks can provide a sense of purpose and accomplishment.

Games and puzzles can be fun ways to stimulate the brain. Choose simple ones like jigsaw puzzles and card games. These activities can help maintain cognitive function and memory.

Storytelling is a powerful tool for memory stimulation. Encourage your loved one to share stories from their past. This activity can provide an opportunity for self-expression and connection.

Physical exercise is known to improve memory and cognitive function. Simple activities like walking or dancing can not only stimulate the brain but also improve overall physical health.

Gardening can be a therapeutic activity. The process of planting, watering, and watching something grow can provide a sense of accomplishment. Plus, the smells and textures can stimulate the senses and evoke memories.

Cooking together can be a bonding activity. Prepare simple recipes that your loved one used to cook. The process can trigger memories and provide an opportunity for conversation.

Emotional and Psychological Support

"The best way to cheer yourself up is to try to cheer somebody else up." - Mark Twain.

Caregiving for a loved one who is living with Alzheimer's or dementia can feel like a lonely road. But you are not alone. It's normal to feel a range of emotions. Let's talk about the emotional and psychological support you need and deserve.

First, self-care is vital. You might think, "But I need to focus on my loved one." True, but think of the safety advice on planes. They tell us to put on our oxygen masks first, then help others. The same applies here. It's not selfish. It's practical. You can't pour from an empty cup.

Next, understand that it's okay to feel. Anger, guilt, sadness, and frustration are common feelings for caregivers. Don't fight them. Accept them. They don't make you a bad person or a bad caregiver. They show that you care.

Remember, it's okay to take a break if you need it. Reach out to others. Talk to friends, family, or a counselor about your feelings. You might worry about burdening them. But sharing your thoughts can lighten your load. It's not weakness. It's part of being human.

Remember, your feelings are valid. It's okay to seek help. It's okay to have bad days. It's okay to feel overwhelmed. But it's also okay to seek joy, laugh, and enjoy time with your loved one.

It's also crucial to stay informed about Alzheimer's and dementia. Knowledge can help reduce fear and stress. It can also help you make informed decisions about your loved one's care. Build a support network. Join a local or online support group. Here, you can share experiences, tips, and encouragement with others who understand your journey. You don't have to face this alone.

Personal Narratives of the Emotional Toll on Families

"A family is a circle of love, not broken by a loss, but made stronger by the memories." - Author Unknown.

Alzheimer's and dementia are hard on everyone. They change the person you love, and they change you too. The emotional toll is often huge. It's a pain that's hard to put into words. No one is ever ready for it.

Families dealing with these conditions face a unique set of challenges. It's a constant cycle of worry and stress about the patient's health, safety, and happiness. The stress of managing their care, keeping them calm, and dealing with the changes in their behavior.

Every day brings a new set of challenges, and every day demands a new level of patience. It's like walking on a tightrope. One wrong step, one moment of lost focus, and everything falls apart.

It's not just the physical strain but the emotional one, too. Seeing your loved one forget their past, forget their memories, and forget who they are is heart-wrenching. It's like losing them piece by piece, day by day. It's a kind of grief that's hard to make sense of.

But amid this pain, there's also love. Love for the person they were, love for the person they are now, and love for the person they're becoming. This love is what keeps families going. It's what helps them find the strength to face each day.

Remember your loved ones have no control over their memory. You may feel like they don't love you because they can't remember you. Although it is difficult and sad, it is important to not take that personally. They can't help it.

Indeed, many families find a new kind of bond in the face of Alzheimer's and dementia. They learn to lean on each other, to find comfort in each other, and to draw strength from each other. They find a new sense of unity amid the chaos and pain.

There are days of joy, too. Days when the patient remembers a precious memory, days when they smile and laugh, days when they're at peace. These moments are rare but worth every bit of the struggle. They remind families of the love that's still there, the love that Alzheimer's and dementia can't take away.

Strategies for Coping with the Emotional Challenges

"In the midst of every crisis lies great opportunity." Albert Einstein

This quote that rings true for you, a caregiver in the throes of Alzheimer's and dementia. You're in a crisis, of course. But there's also an opportunity for growth, development, and profound emotional resilience.

Coping with the emotional challenges of caregiving can feel like a steep mountain. But remember, it's okay to feel what you're feeling. It's normal. It's human. Emotions aren't good or bad. They're just signals, telling us something about our state of mind.

First off, remember self-care. Yes, as a caregiver, you cannot give when you have nothing left to give. You have to take care of yourself, too. Take breaks. Rest. Eat well. Exercise. Do things you love. All these can boost your mood, reduce stress, and help you cope better.

Next, seek support. You're not alone in this. Connect with other caregivers. Share your feelings, fears, and hopes. You'll find comfort, advice, and encouragement in these shared experiences. It's a powerful way to cope, to know that others understand what you're going through. Remember, patience is key. Dealing with Alzheimer's or dementia can be frustrating. But patience helps. It's okay if your loved one forgets names or repeats stories. They're not doing it on purpose. Be patient with them, and be patient with yourself too.

Practice acceptance. This is a tough one, but it helps. Accept the reality of the disease. It's here, and it's not going away. Accepting it doesn't mean giving up. It means facing the challenge head-on and doing your best with what you have.

Mindfulness can be a powerful tool. It's the practice of being present, of focusing on the here and now. It helps reduce stress and anxiety and can boost your mood, too. Try it. Take a few minutes each day to just be. Focus on your breath, on the sounds around you, on the feel of the sun on your skin.

Finally, seek professional help if you need it. If the emotional toll becomes too heavy, don't hesitate to reach out to a mental health professional. There's no shame in it. It's a sign of strength, of knowing when to ask for help.

The Importance of Support Groups and Therapy

"Shared sorrow is half sorrow." - Dutch Proverb.

If you're caring for a loved one with Alzheimer's or dementia, you know it's tough. It's a job you may not have asked for and can feel lonely. You might feel like no one understands what you're going through. But you're not alone. There are others out there, just like you. And they're ready to share their support and wisdom.

Support groups are one way you can connect with these people. They're a place to share your fears and frustrations and get tips and advice. They're also a safe space to express your feelings, which is so essential when dealing with such a challenging task.

But it's not just about the talking. Support groups can also offer resources and information. They can guide you to books, websites, and other tools to help you in your caregiving journey. They can direct you to experts and services providing more specialized help. But most of all, they can give you a sense of community. They can remind you that you're not alone in this.

Therapy is another support tool that can be very helpful. It's a more private space where you can explore your feelings and thoughts. It can help you deal with the stress and anxiety that often come with caregiving. It can also help you manage any feelings of guilt, anger, or grief you might be experiencing.

Therapists are trained to listen and help you find ways to cope. They can help you develop strategies to deal with the challenges you're facing. They can also provide a fresh perspective and help you see things in a new light.

Therapy can also be a place to learn more about Alzheimer's and dementia. Therapists can provide information and resources that can help you understand these conditions better. They can guide you to strategies and techniques to make your caregiving role more manageable.

But the most important thing about therapy is that it's a space just for you. When you're a caregiver, so much of your time and energy goes into caring for someone else. Therapy is a place where you can focus on yourself and your own mental and emotional well-being.

Navigating the Emotional Rollercoaster of Caregiving

"To care for those who once cared for us is one of the highest honors." - Tia Walker.

Being a caregiver is a role filled with both joy and sorrow. It is a role that requires strength and courage. It is also a role that requires patience and love. As a caregiver for a loved one with Alzheimer's or dementia, your strength is tested daily. But you are not alone. This section will help you understand and navigate this emotional rollercoaster.

Taking care of a loved one with Alzheimer's or dementia can be a challenging task. It's not just about the physical care but also the emotional toll it takes. You might often feel overwhelmed, sad, or even angry. These feelings are normal and part of the process.

Remember that your emotions are valid. It's okay to feel upset or frustrated. It's okay to grieve the person your loved one used to be. These feelings don't make you a bad caregiver. They make you human.

Self-care is crucial when you are a caregiver. It's not selfish to take time for yourself. In fact, it's necessary. Regular breaks can help you maintain your emotional health. Find activities that help you relax and recharge. Do something as simple as taking a walk or reading a book.

It's also important to have a support system. This could be family, friends, or a support group. Having people to talk to can help you cope with your feelings. They can provide comfort, advice, and a listening ear when you need it most.

Remember to be kind to yourself. You are doing the best you can in a difficult situation. Don't beat yourself up if you make a mistake or have a bad day. You are human, and it's okay to be imperfect.

You might also find it helpful to learn as much as you can about Alzheimer's and dementia. Understanding these conditions can help you better care for your loved one. It can also help you understand what they are going through.

There are going to be good days and bad days. There will be moments of clarity and moments of confusion. It's important to celebrate the good moments and not dwell on the bad ones.

Patience is critical when caring for a loved one with Alzheimer's or dementia. Their behavior can be unpredictable and sometimes frustrating.

But remember, they are not doing it on purpose. They are dealing with a disease that is changing their brain.

Lessons Learned from Experiences

"Experience is the best teacher, but the tuition is high." - Norwegian proverb.

Alzheimer's and dementia are challenging. They test your resolve and patience. Dealing with these conditions can be a draining ordeal. But it's from these trials that we learn the most.

Your journey as a caregiver is unique. It is filled with ups and downs, moments of joy, and periods of sorrow. However, it's through these varying experiences that we find our strength and resilience. The lessons learned are invaluable, not just for you but for others in similar situations.

The first key lesson is understanding the importance of patience. Alzheimer's and dementia are progressive diseases. They change your loved one's behavior and abilities over time. Patience becomes your greatest ally in these trying times. It helps you weather the storm of changes and difficulties that come with these conditions.

Next, we learn about empathy. Empathy is the ability to understand and share the feelings of another. It's a skill that is honed through time and experience. When you empathize with your loved one, you can better understand their fears and frustrations. It enables you to provide care that is sensitive to their emotional needs.

Another lesson drawn from experience is the necessity of self-care. Caregiving can be exhausting. It can take a toll on your physical and mental well-being. Therefore, it's crucial to take care of yourself. Taking time to rest, relax, and rejuvenate is not selfish. It's essential for you to continue providing the best care to your loved one.

Experience also teaches us to be adaptable. The progression of Alzheimer's and dementia is unpredictable. Your loved one's needs will change, and so should your approach to caregiving. Being flexible and ready to adapt is an important lesson learned through this journey.

Let's not underestimate the importance of support. A strong network of friends, family, support groups and professionals can be a lifeline. They provide a sounding board for your concerns, offer respite when you need a break, and bring fresh perspectives to difficult situations.

From these experiences, we also learn to celebrate small victories. With Alzheimer's and dementia, it's the little moments that matter most. A shared smile, a fond memory recalled, or a peaceful day are all victories. Acknowledging and celebrating these moments bring joy and positivity to the caregiving journey.

You've reached the halfway point of "Empowering Caregivers Through Alzheimer's and Dementia," and I would love to hear what you think.

Your feedback not only helps me, but also fellow caregivers in similar situations.

It' simple to leave a review on Amazon:

Visit the 'Write a Customer Review' page by
or scanning the QR code below
with your mobile phone:

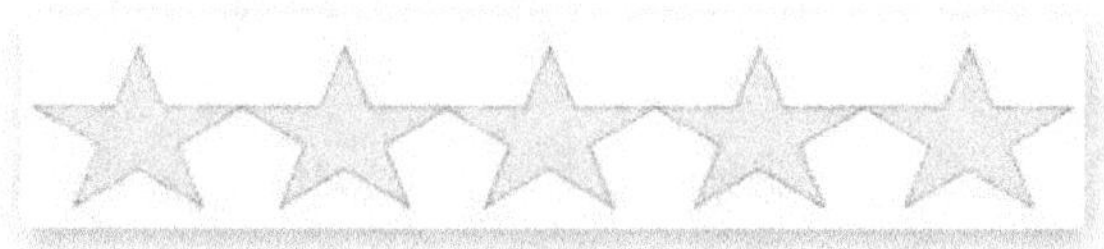

By offering your insights, you're nurturing a collective of caregivers, fostering resilience and solidarity in the face of adversity. Your words can inspire and comfort them, making their caregiving journey easier and more fulfilling. Your thoughts matter. Thank you for being a part of my journey!

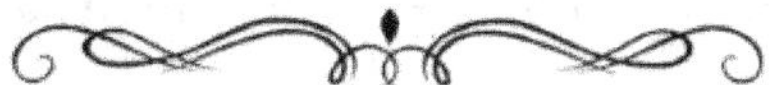

Chapter Five
Creating a Supportive Environment

The best care is home care." - Dorothy Canfield Fisher.

In this section, we'll talk about how you can adapt your home to be dementia-friendly. This is a key step in providing effective care for your loved one with Alzheimer's or dementia.

First of all, safety is a prime concern. Ensuring the home is free from hazards that could lead to falls or injuries is vital. This might involve removing rugs or other trip hazards, installing grab bars in the bathroom, or placing locks on cabinets with dangerous items.

Lighting should also be considered. Well-lit spaces can help prevent confusion and disorientation. Make sure there's plenty of natural light during the day and adequate artificial light at night. Avoid shadows and dark corners as they can create visual illusions that may confuse a person with dementia.

The home should be easy to navigate. Clear pathways and remove clutter. Place essential items in easy-to-find spots. Labeling doors and drawers can also be helpful.

Noise can be a big issue for someone with dementia. Too much noise can lead to agitation or confusion. Try to reduce unnecessary noise as much as possible. This could mean turning off the TV when it's not being watched or using headphones for music.

Keep the home as familiar as possible. Changes in environment can be stressful for someone with dementia. Keep furniture in the same place, and avoid redecorating or moving things around unnecessarily.

Another useful strategy is to create 'activity zones' in the home. These are areas set up for specific tasks or activities and could include a table with art supplies for creative activities or a comfy chair with a basket of books for reading.

Keeping the home clean and tidy is also beneficial. Clutter can lead to confusion and stress. It's also important for hygiene, particularly if the person with dementia has incontinence issues.

It's worth considering some home modifications. For example, you might want to install a walk-in shower or an easy-access toilet. You could also consider safety features such as alarms or sensors that alert you if the person with dementia has a fall or leaves the home.

One final point to consider is the person's personal space. Everyone needs a place where they can retreat and feel safe. This could be a bedroom, a favorite chair, or a spot in the garden. Respect this space and make it as comfortable and inviting as possible.

Adapting Spaces for Loved Ones with Alzheimer's

Living well is an art that can be mastered even in the face of Alzheimer's and dementia. This is a notion that rings true for many families. As caregivers, we hold the power to transform our living spaces to meet the needs of our loved ones. This does not only entail physical changes but also emotional shifts.

The first step is to create a safe environment. Safety is key in any living situation, especially for individuals with Alzheimer's. Simple adjustments can go a long way. Remove objects that can cause trips and falls. Install locks on doors and windows to prevent wandering. Keep medication and cleaning supplies out of reach.

Next, consider the comfort of your loved one. Cozy spaces can help soothe anxiety and confusion. Use soft lighting and calm colors. Keep their favorite items close by. Familiar objects can provide a sense of security and continuity.

Incorporate clear paths and open spaces. Clutter can be overwhelming to a person with Alzheimer's. It can lead to confusion and agitation. Keep furniture to a minimum and ensure clear walking paths, promoting ease of movement and preventing falls.

Visual cues can be beneficial. They can guide your loved one through their daily routine. Use labels for cabinets and drawers. Install signs for bathrooms and bedrooms. Pictures can also be used to identify personal items.

Adapting the living space is one part, but emotional adaptation is equally important. Keep a positive and patient attitude. This can set the tone for the whole household. Understand that your loved one may have good days and bad days. Be flexible and adapt to their changing needs.

Introduce routines and structure. This can provide a sense of predictability for your loved one. It can alleviate anxiety and confusion. Plan activities they enjoy and can safely participate in.

Involve your loved one in daily tasks. This can provide a sense of purpose and involvement. Simple tasks like setting the table or folding laundry can be beneficial. It can boost their self-esteem and give them a sense of accomplishment.

Communication is key in any caregiving situation. Speak clearly and slowly. Use simple words and short sentences. Make sure to maintain eye contact. This can help your loved one focus and understand you better.

Remember to prioritize self-care. Caregiving can be challenging and draining. Taking care of your own physical and emotional health is vital. This ensures you can provide the best care possible for your loved one.

Ensuring Safety and Reducing Potential Hazards

"Safety is not an intellectual exercise to keep us in work. It is a matter of life and death. It is the sum of our contributions to safety management that determines whether the people we work with live or die." - Sir Brian Appleton.

Safety should be a top concern when caring for a loved one with Alzheimer's or dementia. The brain changes that come with these conditions can lead to new behaviors. Some of these can pose risks to your loved one's safety. Let's discuss some ways to ensure safety and reduce potential hazards.

One key aspect of safety is the home environment. Make sure the space is clutter-free, helping prevent falls and other accidents. Keeping paths clear, furniture stable, and rugs secured is best. Check for good lighting as well. This can help your loved one see clearly and avoid tripping over unseen objects.

Managing medication is another important safety aspect. Alzheimer's and dementia can affect a person's ability to remember if they've taken their medication. This can result in missed doses or double dosing. It's vital to help manage their medication. You could use a pill box organizer or set reminders to help with this.

Keeping an eye on kitchen safety is crucial, too. Cooking can be a risk for those with Alzheimer's or dementia. They may forget to turn off the stove or oven. Consider measures like stove locks or automatic shut-off devices. Also, keep sharp objects and cleaning supplies out of reach.

Going on outings can be particularly enjoyable. However it is important to assure that your loved one has on the proper clothing. Too many layers on a hot day can lead to heat exhaustion and not enough clothing on a cold day could lead to hypothermia. Keep in mind, that your loved one may need help with choosing the appropriate attire which will make the adventure fun and stress free.

Another thing to keep in mind is driving safety. Alzheimer's and dementia can affect a person's ability to drive safely. It may be necessary to have a conversation about their driving. This can be a difficult discussion to have. But remember, their safety and the safety of others is the priority.

Wandering is a typical behavior in Alzheimer's and dementia patients. This can be a significant safety concern. Consider installing locks on doors and windows. An identification bracelet can also be helpful, which has their name, your contact info, and their condition noted in it. There are also tracking devices that can be used.

Personal care can pose some risks, too. Alzheimer's and dementia can affect a person's ability to do daily tasks, including bathing, dressing, and grooming. You may need to assist with these tasks. Be patient and give them time to do what they can. They may resist help at times. If so, try to understand their feelings and reassure them.

Fire safety is essential as well. Alzheimer's and dementia can affect a person's judgment. They might not react appropriately in case of a fire. It's a good idea to check smoke detectors regularly. Also, practice fire escape plans with them to prepare them for an emergency.

Safety can also be about preventing abuse. Sadly, those with Alzheimer's and dementia can be targets of scams or abuse. Be vigilant about who has access to your loved one. Monitor their bank accounts and credit cards for signs of fraud.

Establishing Routines and Rituals

"Routine is not a prison, but the way to freedom from time." - May Sarton.

In the care of Alzheimer's and dementia patients, having a routine is a powerful tool. It provides a structure that brings comfort to both the caregiver and the one receiving care. The world can seem less chaotic and more familiar when there are routines to follow.

Routines offer a sense of control. When things become blurry for dementia patients, having a set schedule provides needed clarity. It is a beacon of stability in the ever-changing fog of their cognitive abilities.

There is a calming effect in knowing what comes next. Uncertainty can be a source of anxiety for dementia patients. With a routine, the element of surprise is minimized, leading to a decrease in behavioral issues often associated with Alzheimer's and dementia.

Predictability is a cushion amidst the confusion. Regular routines provide a comforting pattern that can help reduce agitation and improve overall well-being. Daily activities such as meals, bathing, and bedtime can serve as anchors, providing a sense of security amidst the uncertainty that dementia often brings.

Repetition is a friend, not a foe, in this context. For someone with Alzheimer's, the familiar is comforting. Regular activity can help maintain their abilities and encourage a sense of accomplishment. Routines are not merely schedules but rituals that bring meaning to everyday life. They can be as simple as a morning cup of tea or a nightly bedtime story. These rituals can foster connections, evoke memories, and bring joy to the caregiver and the loved one.

However, it's important to tailor routines to the individual. What works for one person may not work for another. A person's background, interests, and physical capabilities should all be considered when establishing routines. This personalized approach can make the routines more enjoyable and effective.

Flexibility is also essential. Routines should not be rigid. If a loved one is having a bad day or an activity is causing distress, making adjustments is okay. The key is to maintain a balance between structure and adaptability.

Incorporating routines and rituals can make the caregiving journey smoother. They offer a predictable structure that can reduce anxiety and improve quality of life. But remember, each person is unique. The goal is to create a routine that provides comfort, reduces anxiety, and enhances the well-being of your loved one.

So, as you navigate this path, remember the power of routine. It's not just about keeping time; it's about creating a comforting rhythm in a world that often feels out of sync. When done right, routines can be a source of stability in the unpredictable world of Alzheimer's and dementia care.

Stories of Successful Caregiving Routines

"Caregiving, like any other significant task, requires a routine that is both caring and effective." - Author Unknown.

In the world of caregiving, routine is key. Those with Alzheimer's and dementia find comfort in the familiar. They favor the known over the unknown. This is why setting a successful caregiving routine can make a world of difference.

The power of routine lies in its ability to create a sense of safety and predictability. For someone with Alzheimer's or dementia, the world can often seem confusing and uncertain. A solid routine can help alleviate this feeling.

So, what does a successful caregiving routine look like? It's built around the needs and preferences of the person with dementia. This can include their favorite meals, activities they enjoy, and times they prefer to rest.

A good routine starts with the basics. Make sure meals are served at the same time every day. This helps to regulate the body's internal clock and can improve sleep patterns. It's also important to include regular times for personal care, such as bathing and dressing.

In addition to the basics, it's crucial to include stimulating activities in the routine. This can be anything from a walk in the park to a simple puzzle. Such activities can keep the mind active and engaged.

Remember to be flexible in your routine. While routine is important, it's equally important to be able to adapt when necessary. For instance, if the person with dementia is having a particularly bad day, it might be best to skip some activities and focus on providing comfort instead.

While establishing a routine can be helpful, it's also essential to remember that what works for one person may not work for another. Each person with Alzheimer's or dementia is unique, and their routine should be tailored to their individual needs and preferences.

A successful caregiving routine is also one that considers the caregiver's needs. Caring for someone with Alzheimer's or dementia can be physically and emotionally draining. It's critical to build in time for rest and self-care. One key to a successful caregiving routine is consistency. Once you've established a routine, stick to it as closely as possible. This can provide a sense of security and predictability for the person with dementia.

Communicating the routine to other family members or caregivers is also essential. This ensures that everyone is on the same page and can help to maintain a sense of consistency.

Another aspect of a successful caregiving routine involves monitoring and adjusting as necessary. Over time, the needs of the person with dementia may change. Being observant and willing to adjust the routine as needed is important.

The Significance of Meaningful Rituals

"Rituals are the formulas by which harmony is restored." - Terry Tempest Williams.

The role of rituals can't be ignored when caring for loved ones with Alzheimer's or dementia. More than habits, rituals hold deep meaning. They offer comfort and a sense of order in what can feel like a world turned upside down.

Let's start with an example. Picture a Sunday night family dinner. It's a ritual in many homes. The food on the table might change, but the people, the time, and the laughter stay the same. For someone with dementia, this ritual can be a tether, a link to the familiar.

When memory ebbs, rituals can fill the void. The scent of a particular dish and the sound of family chatter, these sensory cues spark deep, emotional memories. They may not recall the details, but the feeling of being loved and of belonging remains.

This is the power of meaningful rituals. They can help your loved one connect to the past and their identity. Rituals can offer some semblance of control in a world where memory is fleeting.

Now, it's important to note that not all rituals are created equal. What works for one person might not work for another. The key lies in finding those rituals that hold meaning for your loved one. It could be as simple as a nightly cup of tea or as involved as a weekly family gathering.

You might be wondering how to identify these rituals. Start by recalling the routines your loved one enjoyed before their diagnosis. Did they have a favorite park for walks? A preferred breakfast spot? These can be transformed into meaningful rituals.

The beauty of rituals lies in their flexibility. If your loved one's health declines, you can adapt the ritual. The park walk might become a drive, and the breakfast out might become a meal in. The essence of the ritual remains, even as the details change.

It's also worth noting that these rituals are not just for your loved one. They can be a source of comfort for you, the caregiver, as well. Amid the daily demands of caregiving, rituals can offer a chance to breathe and find joy in the moment.

The benefits of rituals are rooted in science. Research shows that familiar routines can reduce anxiety in individuals with dementia. They can also improve sleep patterns and overall mood.

But more than just the physiological benefits, rituals offer a deeper connection. They can open a window into the world of your loved one, a world that might seem closed off due to their condition. Through these rituals, you can reach out, hold their hand, and let them know they are not alone.

Creating meaningful rituals won't erase the challenges of Alzheimer's or dementia. But they can offer moments of clarity, of connection, amidst the fog. They can remind your loved one and you of the love that endures beyond memory loss.

Day-to-Day Activities: Engaging Activities to Stimulate Cognition

"The heart, like the mind, has a memory. And in it are kept the most precious keepsakes." - Henry Wadsworth Longfellow.

An essential part of being a caregiver for a loved one with Alzheimer's or dementia is finding ways to engage them mentally. Stimulating activities can help slow cognitive decline, keep your loved one engaged, and provide a meaningful way for you to connect with them.

One simple yet effective activity is looking at old photos. This can help spark memories and lead to interesting conversations. It's also a great way to keep your loved one's past alive and valued. You'll be surprised at the stories that can come from a single photograph.

Music, too, can be a powerful stimulus. Research shows that music can reach parts of the brain that other forms of communication cannot. Create a playlist of their favorite songs from the past. Sing along or even get up and dance if they are able. These simple activities can bring joy and a sense of connection.

Simple puzzles and games can also be beneficial. Choose games familiar to your loved one, such as a simple card game they used to play or a crossword puzzle, making sure the game is at a level they can handle to avoid frustration.

Reading together is another engaging activity. Choose books that your loved one enjoyed in the past. If reading is difficult for them, you can read aloud. This can be a soothing activity and a great way to bond.

Cooking together can also be a stimulating activity. Involve your loved one in simple tasks like stirring or sorting ingredients, helping them feel helpful and engaged. Plus, it's a great way to enjoy a meal together. Gardening is another activity that can be beneficial. The act of planting and caring for plants can be therapeutic. Consider indoor plants or a window box if an outdoor garden isn't possible.

Simple crafts can also be a fun way to engage your loved one. Choose crafts that are within their ability level, like making a scrapbook, painting, or knitting. The act of creating something can bring a sense of accomplishment and joy.

Physical activity is also essential, perhaps taking a simple walk around the block or doing gentle yoga. Please make sure any physical activity is approved by their doctor.

Creative Ideas for Spending Quality Time Together

"The best thing to hold onto in life is each other." - Audrey Hepburn.

As caregivers, we know the unique challenges Alzheimer's and dementia present. It can be tough to connect with our loved ones in ways we once did. But worry not. There are creative ways to spend time together to enhance bonds and bring joy.

Remember, it's not about the grand scale of the activities but rather the quality of the moments shared. The first idea is to create a memory box. This box can be filled with items that spark memories from their past. Photos, music records, or even trinkets from a favorite vacation can trigger meaningful conversations.

Secondly, consider music therapy. Music has a profound impact on our brains. It can help recall memories and emotions. Make a playlist of their favorite songs and enjoy them together. Singing along or dancing can also be a fun way to interact.

Next, try gardening. Gardening is a calming activity that can be done together. It can provide a sense of achievement and satisfaction. Whether planting flowers or vegetables, it's a wonderful way to spend the day.

Cooking together can be another engaging activity. Recreate recipes that they once loved. The smell and taste of familiar foods can stimulate memories and conversations.

Art therapy is another powerful way to connect. It can be as simple as coloring or as complex as painting. Artistic expression can help in expressing feelings that words cannot.

Reading is another activity that can be beneficial. Read out loud their favorite books or newspapers. It not only keeps them informed but also stimulates their cognitive skills.

Lastly, the simple act of taking a walk can be therapeutic. A stroll in the park or around the neighborhood can provide fresh air and a change of scenery. Remember to make these walks slow and relaxing.

These activities may not always go as planned. There might be days when your loved one is unresponsive or agitated. It's important to be patient and flexible. What matters most is the connection and the shared moments. While these activities are beneficial, it's crucial to consider the person's current abilities and preferences. It's not about filling the day with activities but rather about finding those that bring the most joy and comfort.

It's also important to remember that as a caregiver, you must take care of yourself. Take time to refresh and recharge. Self-care is not selfish; it's necessary.

These activities are not only for the person with Alzheimer's or dementia. They are also for you, the caregiver. They are opportunities to connect, to understand, and to love. Let these shared moments remind you of the bond you share beyond the confines of memory loss.

The Therapeutic Value of Music, Art, and Sensory Experiences

"Music can change the world because it can change people." - Bono.

This quote from a world-famous singer holds true. Music, art, and sensory experiences can do wonders, especially for those living with Alzheimer's and dementia.

In the realm of Alzheimer's care, the use of music is profound. Music therapy can unlock memories and kickstart the grey matter. It's a way for your loved ones to reconnect with the world. Studies show that music can improve mood, reduce stress, and even reduce symptoms of Alzheimer's.

Art, too, has a powerful impact. Art therapy can provide a sense of accomplishment. It's a way for your loved ones to express themselves when words fail. Art can bring joy, stimulate the mind, and improve overall well-being.

Sensory experiences also play a role in Alzheimer's care. Things like touch, smell, and taste can trigger memories. Simple activities like baking a familiar recipe can bring comfort. Or a soft blanket may provide a sense of security.

Let's delve into these therapies a bit more. You'll see how they can bring joy and peace to your loved ones.

Music therapy is a hit in Alzheimer's care. Why? Studies show that our brains are hard-wired to connect music with long-term memory. Even for persons with severe dementia, music can tap deep emotional recall. Music can provide a way back for individuals who have lost the ability to connect with the world. And music can have a calming effect on a restless or agitated person.

But how do you use music therapy? Start simple. Play songs from your loved one's youth. You'll be amazed at the memories it can stir. Sing along, dance, or just enjoy the music. You can also try playing soothing music. It can reduce agitation and improve sleep.

Art therapy is another tool in our kit. It's a way for your loved ones to express their feelings. When words are hard to find, art can speak. It allows for self-expression and communication. It can reduce feelings of isolation. It's also a great way to relax.

How can you use art therapy? Provide a range of materials - from paints to clay. Let your loved one create. Don't worry about the end product. It's the process that's important. You could also try coloring books. They're a fun and easy way to engage.

Sensory experiences are also so vital. Our senses are linked to memory. A familiar scent or taste can bring back memories. It can provide comfort and spark conversation.

How can you use sensory experiences? Try cooking a favorite meal. Or use scented lotions during a massage. Even a walk in the garden can stir memories.

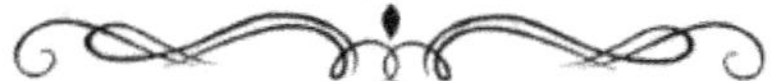

Chapter Six
Nutrition and Well-Being

It's no secret that food plays a crucial role in our health. But did you know it can also impact our brain health? Yes, it's true. A balanced diet can do wonders for the brain, especially when dealing with conditions like Alzheimer's and dementia.

Now, you might ask, "What does a balanced diet look like?" It's a fair question. In simple terms, a balanced diet includes a mix of proteins, carbs, fats, vitamins, and minerals. It's about eating a wide range of foods to get the nutrients your body needs.

But how does this link to brain health? Well, studies have shown that certain nutrients can protect the brain. For example, omega-3 fatty acids aid in brain function. Foods rich in antioxidants, like fruits and veggies, can also help protect the brain.

Don't just take our word for it. Listen to the experts. We've spoken with nutritionists who specialize in Alzheimer's and dementia. They agree that a balanced diet can significantly impact brain health.

One nutritionist shared a story about a patient named Mary. Mary was in the early stages of Alzheimer's. The nutritionist suggested some dietary changes. The focus was on whole foods and cutting out processed items.

Mary's family saw changes after a few months. Mary seemed more alert. Her memory seemed to improve. Of course, diet wasn't the only factor. However, the family felt it played a role in Mary's improvement.

Stories like Mary's are not rare. Many people have seen improvements after dietary changes. But remember, it's not a one-size-fits-all. What works for one person may not work for another.

The key is to find what works for you and your loved one. It might take some trial and error. But don't be discouraged. The journey to better brain health through nutrition is a marathon, not a sprint.

That said, it's crucial not to overlook the role of a balanced diet. It's an essential piece of the puzzle. And it's something we all have control over. We can choose what we put into our bodies. And by making wise choices, we can support our brain health.

Exercise and Physical Health

"The body achieves what the mind believes." This is so true, especially when it comes to caring for loved ones with Alzheimer's and dementia.

Physical activity plays a crucial role in our overall health. More so, it has a significant effect on our cognitive function. Regular exercise can help improve memory and attention and even slow down cognitive decline in Alzheimer's patients. This might seem surprising, but recent studies corroborate this claim.

Research shows that regular exercise can improve brain health. It boosts blood flow to the brain, which delivers essential nutrients. In turn, this helps maintain healthy brain cells and encourages the growth of new ones.

Now, you may wonder how to incorporate exercise into your caregiving routine. This can be daunting, especially if your loved one isn't used to being active. But don't worry, starting small is key.

For instance, a simple walk in the park can be a good start. It's a low-impact activity that can be easily adjusted to suit your loved one's physical abilities. Plus, it's an excellent opportunity to spend quality time together, enjoy nature, and get fresh air.

In addition, you can try chair exercises. These are exercises that can be done while sitting down. They're perfect for individuals with mobility issues. Chair exercises can improve flexibility, strength, and cardiac health.

Another option could be water-based exercises. If your loved one enjoys swimming, this could be an excellent choice. Water-based exercises are gentle on the joints and can improve muscle strength.

Aside from the physical benefits, exercise also plays a vital role in mental health. It helps reduce stress, anxiety, and feelings of depression. This can immensely improve the quality of life for your loved one.

However, it's important to note that you should always consult a healthcare professional before starting any new exercise regimen to ensure the activities are safe and suitable for your loved one's health.

Now, keeping a loved one with Alzheimer's or dementia active might seem like an arduous task. You might face resistance or reluctance from them. But don't lose heart.

Make the activities enjoyable and engaging. You can do this by incorporating things they love into the activities. If they enjoy music, play their favorite songs during exercise time. If they love nature, take them for walks in the park or garden.

Patience and understanding are essential in this journey. There might be days when they don't feel like doing anything. And that's okay. The goal is not to push them but to gently encourage them to stay active and healthy.

Mindfulness and Stress Reduction

Caregiving is not just about the physical tasks. It's also about the mental and emotional well-being of both the caregiver and the patient. In this section, we will explore the importance of mindfulness, its role in stress reduction, and how it can lead to better caregiving outcomes. Remember, a peaceful caregiver creates a relaxed environment for the patient.

"Mindfulness is the miracle by which we master and restore ourselves." - Thich Nhat Hanh.

Mindfulness is a tool that can help caregivers navigate the stormy seas of Alzheimer's and dementia care. It might seem like a buzzword, but it's a time-proven practice that can lead to inner peace amidst the chaos. It's not a magic pill but a skill that needs to be honed and used.

Mindfulness can start with simple practices. For instance, paying attention to your breath can help anchor you in the present moment. Try to focus on your breathing for a few minutes each day. Feel the air entering and leaving your body. It's a simple yet powerful technique to calm your mind and body.

Another mindfulness technique is to focus on your senses. What can you hear? What can you see? What can you smell? By honing in on your senses, you can root yourself in the present moment and reduce feelings of stress and anxiety.

There are countless stories of caregivers who have found inner peace amidst the chaos. They speak of the transformation that mindfulness has brought into their lives. These caregivers have learned to pause, breathe, and respond rather than react. They have found a sanctuary of calm within the storm.

Mindfulness doesn't stop at the caregiver. It has a ripple effect. When you, as a caregiver, are calm and present, it can positively impact the person you are caring for. Your peace and calm can help instill the same feelings in your loved one. Remember, emotions can be contagious.

The connection between caregiver well-being and patient well-being is well-documented. Research has shown that when caregivers are less stressed and care for their mental health, it can lead to better patient outcomes. This is particularly true in Alzheimer's and dementia care, where the emotional state of the caregiver can significantly influence the patient's mood and behavior.

Mindfulness is not a cure-all but a valuable tool in a caregiver's toolbox. It can provide a respite, however brief, from the pressures of caregiving. It can help you stay present and focused, making you a better caregiver.

In the end, mindfulness is about compassion. It's about being kind to yourself and your loved one. It's about recognizing that amid the storm, there is a calm center. And in that calm center, you can find the strength and resilience to continue on this caregiving journey.

Chapter Seven
Advanced Care and Hospice

"The ultimate test of a moral society is the kind of world that it leaves to its children." - Dietrich Bonhoeffer.

When the time comes to transition a loved one into advanced care, it is often a period of high emotional stress. Many families grapple with this tough decision, fraught with a mix of love, pain, and a sense of responsibility. The stories of such families can serve as a guiding light for others in a similar situation.

During these emotional storms, the first step often involves identifying the proper care facility. This is not always an easy task. It requires a careful balance of evaluating the quality of care, the facility's reputation, and the needs of your loved one. One essential tip is to be thorough, ask plenty of questions, and visit multiple facilities before making a decision.

It is also important to remember that each facility is different. Some focus on physical health, while others prioritize mental well-being. The right choice depends on the unique needs of your loved one. Therefore, it is crucial to clearly understand these needs before embarking on the search.

Making the difficult decision to transition a loved one to a care facility is an emotional journey. It can be a time of profound sadness, as you may feel a sense of loss. However, it is essential to remember that this decision is often the best choice for your loved one's well-being.

It is also a time of adjustment. The change in environment, routine, and caregivers can be overwhelming for your loved one. It is common for them to experience feelings of fear, confusion, or resistance. As a caregiver, your role is to provide reassurance and emotional support during this transition.

One way to do this is by maintaining open and honest communication. Talk to your loved one about the transition, what to expect, and why it is happening. Open communication can help alleviate some of their fears and anxieties.

Another critical aspect of the transition process is patience. Change is hard, especially for those with Alzheimer's or dementia. It takes time for them to adjust to a new environment and routine. Therefore, patience and understanding are crucial during this period.

In addition, it is essential for caregivers to take care of their personal emotional health during this transition. It is normal to feel a range of emotions, from guilt and sadness to relief and hope. Seek support from friends, family, or support groups if needed.

Hospice and End-of-Life Care

"The last stages of life can be very rich and fulfilling, with opportunities to mend fences, make amends, and say good-bye." - Maggie Callanan and Patricia Kelley, Final Gifts: Understanding the Special Awareness, Needs, and Communications of the Dying.

Hospice care plays a vital role when it comes to Alzheimer's and dementia. It focuses on comfort rather than cure, providing physical, psychological, and spiritual support for those in the final stages of life. This type of care aims to improve the quality of life for the patient, even when their condition is no longer curable. It provides relief from pain and other symptoms, helping the person live as fully and comfortably as possible.

Navigating end-of-life decisions can be a challenging task for families. It's a time filled with emotional turmoil but also an opportunity for closure. Sharing personal narratives can provide a sense of connection and understanding. These stories can offer comfort, providing a roadmap for those facing similar situations. They show that while every journey is unique, there are shared experiences and common emotions that can bring us together.

Finding comfort during this stage is essential. It's a time for reflection, for cherishing memories, and for saying goodbyes. It's about making the most of the time left, ensuring that the person's final days are filled with love and dignity, including spending quality time together, reminiscing about shared experiences, and expressing love and gratitude.

Closure is an essential aspect of end-of-life care. It offers a way to say goodbye, to express love and gratitude, and to come to terms with the impending loss. Closure can take many forms, from discussions about the person's life and legacy to more formal rituals or ceremonies. The goal is to provide a sense of peace and acceptance for the person nearing the end of their life and their loved ones.

Hospice care can be a valuable resource during this time, providing medical care to manage symptoms and improve comfort, as well as emotional and spiritual support. The hospice team can also offer guidance and support to family members, helping them navigate end-of-life decisions and cope with their grief.

The role of hospice care in Alzheimer's and dementia goes beyond medical treatment. It encompasses a holistic approach that considers the person's physical, emotional, and spiritual needs. It's about enhancing the quality of life, providing comfort, and ensuring dignity in the final stages of life.

As caregivers, it's essential to understand and embrace the role of hospice care. It's not about giving up but rather about providing the best possible care in the final stages of life and focusing on comfort, quality of life, and dignity rather than cure.

Sharing personal narratives can provide a sense of connection and understanding. These stories can offer comfort, providing a roadmap for those facing similar situations. They show that while every journey is unique, there are shared experiences and common emotions that can bring us together.

Navigating end-of-life decisions can be challenging. It's a time of emotional turmoil but also an opportunity for closure. Open and honest discussions help clarify the person's wishes, ensuring their values and preferences guide their care.

Finding comfort and closure during this stage is crucial. It's a time for reflection, for cherishing memories, and for saying goodbyes. It's about making the most of the time left, ensuring that the person's final days are filled with love and dignity.

Closure is an essential part of end-of-life care. It provides a way to say goodbye, to express love and gratitude, and to come to terms with the impending loss; and about finding peace and acceptance, both for the person nearing the end of their life and for their loved ones.

In conclusion, hospice care plays a critical role in Alzheimer's and dementia, providing comfort and support in the final stages of life. Navigating end-of-life decisions can be challenging, but sharing personal narratives can provide guidance and comfort.

Ultimately, the goal is to find comfort and closure during this stage, cherishing the time left and ensuring dignity and peace in the person's final days.

Chapter Eight
Legal and Ethical Considerations

"If the law has made you a witness, remain a man of science. You have no victim to avenge, no guilty or innocent person to ruin or save. You must bear testimony within the limits of science." - Dr. Paul Brouardel.

As caregivers for persons with Alzheimer's or dementia, it's crucial to understand the legal side of things. Knowing this helps you make better choices for your loved ones. It also protects them and you from legal issues that might come up.

Legal documents are vitally important. They ensure that the wishes of your loved ones are honored and their rights are upheld. These documents could include wills, powers of attorney, and healthcare directives.

A will is a legal paper. It states who will get your loved one's property after they pass away. A power of attorney lets someone make decisions for your loved one when they can't. A healthcare directive outlines your loved one's wishes for medical care if they can't tell the doctor themselves. The most popular and most widely used advance directives for health care are the living will and the durable power of attorney for health care.

It's crucial to have these documents ready. The time will come when your loved one can no longer make decisions. Having these documents can ensure that their wishes are carried out.

One very important legal matter that is often overlooked is to verify that beneficiaries on all investments, retirement accounts, life insurance policies, etc are current and consistent with the will. Altering these after your loved one is unable to make decisions can be costly and difficult.

The legal aspects of Alzheimer's and dementia care can be overwhelming. But they are critical. Laws can vary from state to state and country to country. Learn what the laws are in your area that apply to your loved one's care. Work with a lawyer to make sure you're doing everything right if financially possible.

There are many additional legal challenges in Alzheimer's and dementia care. These might include issues with care costs, property rights, and treatment decisions. But remember, there are also solutions to these challenges.

For instance, a family might struggle to pay for their loved one's care. Financial aid is available for those who qualify. Some families might have a trust fund to help cover costs.

Let's look at another example. A person with dementia may be unable to make decisions about their property. But, with a power of attorney in place, a trusted financial agent could make these decisions for them. This helps protect the person's property and ensures that their wishes are upheld.

These are just a few examples. There are many more legal challenges and solutions in Alzheimer's and dementia care. However, knowing what to do and having the proper legal documents in place make the decision-making process much more manageable. It can also help you provide the best care for your loved one.

Ethical Dilemmas

"Ethics is knowing the difference between what you have a right to do and what is right to do." - Potter Stewart.

Caregiving for a loved one with Alzheimer's or dementia is not a simple task. It's filled with tough choices and ethical dilemmas. You're in a place where you must make decisions for another person. The burden can seem immense.

To begin, let's talk about the concept of ethical dilemmas. In intricate scenarios, you might find yourself confronted with the need to choose between conflicting options, all of which may appear justifiable, yet necessitating the selection of just one. For instance, a common ethical dilemma in caregiving arises when a loved one refuses to move to a memory care facility. They don't want to leave their home and be away from their family. But allowing them to remain is unsafe. What do you do?

Ethical dilemmas are not only challenging but can also lead to stress. You might feel guilty or worried about your choices. This is normal. But remember, there is no perfect answer. You're doing the best you can in a tough situation.

Now, let's talk about some stories of families who faced these tough decisions. These are real people, just like you, who had to make hard choices.

One story is about a woman named Mary. Her mom had Alzheimer's and lived with her. Mary's mom would often wander off and get lost. Mary had to decide if she should lock the doors and risk her mom getting upset or keep them open and risk her mom getting hurt.

Another story is about a man named John. His dad had dementia and would forget to eat. John had to choose between forcing his dad to eat and respecting his dad's choices.

These stories show how hard these choices can be. But they also show that you're not alone. Many caregivers face these same dilemmas.

So, how do we approach and resolve these dilemmas? There is no one-size-fits-all answer. But there are some steps you can take.

First, know your loved one's wishes. If they were able to make the decision, what would they want? This might not always be clear, but it's a great place to start.

Second, get advice. Talk to doctors, nurses, or social workers. They can give you a medical point of view.

Third, take care of yourself. If you're stressed and tired, it will be harder to make good decisions. So, make sure you're getting the rest and support you need.

Lastly, don't be too hard on yourself. As we said before, these are tough choices. You're doing the best you can. And that's all anyone can ask for.

In the end, being a caregiver is about love. It's about doing what's best for your loved one, even when it's hard. It's about respect, dignity, and kindness. It's about making tough choices and doing the best you can. And that's what makes you a fantastic caregiver.

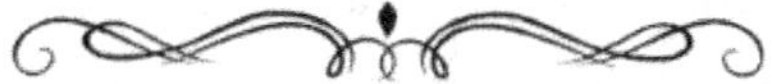

Chapter Nine
The Impact on Family Dynamics
and Planning

"Families are the compass that guides us. They are the inspiration to reach great heights, and our comfort when we occasionally falter." - Brad Henry.

Let's take a moment to talk about sibling relationships. Alzheimer's caregiving can often strain these bonds. We've heard personal accounts from many caregivers. They tell us how the role has influenced their relations with brothers and sisters. Some see a rift growing. Others find it brings them closer. All agree it changes the dynamics.

There's a common thread in these stories. Caregiving puts a spotlight on old patterns and roles. The eldest may still be seen as the responsible one. The youngest might still be viewed as the baby. But Alzheimer's care demands that everyone step up. It asks us to let go of old roles and find new ways to connect.

It can be challenging. But it's possible. And it starts with communication. Open, honest, and frequent discussions can help maintain unity. You can share your feelings, your fears, and your needs. You can also listen. Hear what your siblings have to say. Understand their perspective. It might be different from yours, but it's just as valid.

Strategies for maintaining unity are many. They range from regular family meetings to shared caregiving duties. Even carving out some fun time together can make a difference. Remember, you're not just caregivers. You're brothers and sisters, too. You share a history. You share memories. And now, you share a mission.

Let's move on to cooperation, which is very critical in Alzheimer's care. Everyone needs to pull together. Tasks need to be divided. Decisions need to be made. And everyone's input is valuable. Cooperation means working together towards a common goal. That goal is the best possible care for your loved one.

We often hear stories of families coming together during challenging times. Alzheimer's certainly qualifies. It's a test, no doubt. But it's also an excellent opportunity to strengthen your bonds, to deepen your love, and to show your commitment. You're not just caring for a loved one with Alzheimer's. You're caring for each other too.

It's inspiring to see families rise to the challenge. To witness brothers and sisters becoming a team. To see old grudges give way to new understanding. To watch as the shared goal of caregiving brings them closer. These are the stories that give us hope. They show us what's possible.

In closing, remember this. You're not alone. You have each other. Together, you have the power to make a difference, provide the best possible care for your loved one, and maintain the family unity and cooperation that is essential in this journey. Yes, Alzheimer's changes everything. But it doesn't have to break your bonds. In fact, it can make them stronger.

Invest in your sibling relationships. They're worth it. They are your allies in this fight. They're your support system. They're your family. And together, you can navigate the challenges of Alzheimer's caregiving. You can find the strength you didn't know you had. You can make a difference in your loved one's life. And in the process, you might just find that you've made a difference in your own life, too.

Spousal Caregiving

"Love does not consist of gazing at each other, but in looking outward together in the same direction." - Antoine de Saint-Exupery.

When a spouse is diagnosed with Alzheimer's or dementia, the bonds of marriage are put to the test. It's a shift from being partners to becoming a caregiver. This change can be a hard pill to swallow. Yet, many spouses take up this role with love and dedication. Their stories are filled with resilience, courage, and unwavering commitment.

These stories often highlight the emotional toll of caregiving. Watching a loved one's memories fade can be heart-wrenching. It stirs an emotional storm of sadness, anger, guilt, and even resentment. It's normal to feel a sense of loss. The spouse you knew seems to be fading away, replaced by someone who may not even recognize you.

Coping with these emotional challenges requires inner strength and resilience. It's crucial to remember that it's okay to feel these emotions.

They don't make you a bad spouse or caregiver. It's a part of the process. Accepting these feelings can be the first step to dealing with them effectively.

One strategy that has proven helpful is seeking support. Whether it's a support group, therapy, or simply sharing with friends and family, expressing your feelings can lighten the burden. It's also essential to take care of your own health. A healthy body can support a healthy mind, better equipping you to deal with emotional stress.

Balancing caregiving and maintaining a marriage can be a tightrope walk. The demands of caregiving can overshadow the needs of the marriage, and the marital dynamics change. Conversations revolve around care plans and medical appointments. This shift can make the relationship feel more clinical than romantic.

Yet, it's crucial for spousal caregivers to remember they are still in a marriage. Finding moments to connect beyond the caregiving role can help. Simple acts such as holding hands, sharing a meal, or reminiscing about happy memories can make a huge difference. Even if your spouse doesn't remember these moments, the emotional connection can still exist and provide comfort.

Maintaining personal interests and activities outside of caregiving is essential, providing a much-needed break and a chance to recharge. It can also remind you of your individual identity beyond being a caregiver.

Caring for a spouse with Alzheimer's or dementia is a journey filled with challenges. But amidst the hardships, there are stories of incredible love and resilience. These stories serve as a beacon of hope and a testament to the power of commitment. They remind us that the heart remembers even in the face of memory loss.

Grandchildren and Caregiving

"There is a garden in every childhood, an enchanted place where colors are brighter, the air softer, and the morning more fragrant than ever again." - Elizabeth Lawrence.

Grandkids hold a special place. They see life through a lens of wonder and curiosity. When they turn into caregivers, it's a new role. It's a role that profoundly shapes them and creates bonds that last a lifetime.

The role of a grandchild as a caregiver is unique. They see their grandparent with love and respect. They also see the changes that Alzheimer's brings. It's a challenging role but also one filled with love and understanding.

Some grandkids have shared their stories. They talk about the joys and the trials. They discuss the way they have learned to care for their loved one. It's a journey that has taught them about patience, kindness, and the value of every moment.

The role of a caregiver is a tough one. It requires sacrifice and strength. But these grandkids have shown that it's a role they are willing to take on. They do it with grace and dignity, showing the depth of their love for their grandparent.

These interviews give us insight into their world. They show us the impact of Alzheimer's. They also show us the power of love and resilience. These stories are a testament to the strength of these young caregivers.

Intergenerational caregiving affects family bonds. It strengthens them. It creates a deep connection between grandparent and grandchild. This connection is a powerful one, one that transcends the challenges of Alzheimer's.

Being a caregiver is very demanding. But it's also a role that gives back so much. It's a role that teaches about love, patience, and the power of human connection. It's a role that shapes a person in profound ways.

The grandchildren who take on this role are inspiring. They show us what it means to love unconditionally. They show us the power of resilience. They are a testament to the strength and courage of the human spirit.

Chapter Ten
Looking Ahead with Hope

"The future can be better than the present, and I have the power to make it so." -
Dr. David Burns.

The world of Alzheimer's and dementia research is a domain of constant change. Every day, scientists and doctors work to uncover more about these conditions. They aim to improve treatments and, ultimately, find a cure. This quest for knowledge is a beacon of hope for millions worldwide.

Research and Advancements

In recent years, research on Alzheimer's and dementia has made great strides. Scientists have been focusing on understanding the root causes of these conditions. They delve into the molecular biology of the brain, exploring how and why cells degenerate. Their findings pave the way for new and more effective treatments.

Clinical trials are a vital part of this research. They test the safety and effectiveness of potential treatments. These trials involve real people, including patients and healthy volunteers. Families, too, often play a critical role. Participating in a clinical trial can be a way of fighting back against Alzheimer's and dementia. It's a chance to contribute to the search for a cure.

The stories of families participating in clinical trials are both moving and inspiring. They highlight the human side of Alzheimer's and dementia research. These families face an uncertain future with courage and resilience. They offer a powerful reminder of why this research matters.

New treatments are on the horizon thanks to these efforts. Some aim to slow the progression of Alzheimer's and dementia. Others hope to halt it altogether. While a cure is not yet available, these advancements are a significant step forward. They provide hope to patients and their families.

Caring for someone with Alzheimer's or dementia can be a daunting task. But it's important to remember that you're not alone. A whole community of caregivers is out there, sharing their experiences and offering support. There are also numerous resources available, from educational materials to support groups.

The future of Alzheimer's and dementia care is promising. Research is leading to better treatments and support strategies. It's also shedding light on how to prevent these conditions in the first place. This progress is a testament to the power of science and the human spirit. It's a source of hope for all those affected by Alzheimer's and dementia.

As we look to the future, there's reason to be optimistic. The pace of research is accelerating. Every day brings us closer to understanding these conditions and finding a cure. This progress is due, in large part, to the tireless efforts of scientists, doctors, and families. Their dedication is an inspiration to us all.

To all caregivers out there, remember this: Your work is invaluable. Your compassion and dedication make a difference every day. You're part of a significant effort to fight Alzheimer's and dementia. Together, we can look forward to a future where these conditions are no longer a source of fear and uncertainty.

In this fight, hope is our most powerful weapon. It drives us to keep going, even in the face of adversity. It's what fuels the quest for a cure. And it's what keeps us believing in a better future. Because no matter how difficult the journey, we know that every step forward brings us closer to our goal.

So, let's look ahead with hope. Let's believe in the power of research and advancements. Let's stand together in the face of Alzheimer's and dementia. And let's keep striving for a future where these conditions are a thing of the past. Because together, we can make a difference. Together, we can change the future.

Building a Legacy

"To care for those who once cared for us is one of the highest honors." - Tia Walker.

Building a legacy is about more than just leaving money or property to your loved ones. It's about leaving a lasting impact on their lives, shaping their values, and influencing their future in meaningful ways. For caregivers of Alzheimer's and dementia patients, this legacy often comes in the form of caregiving itself. The skills, empathy, and resilience developed while caring for a loved one can be a powerful legacy that impacts future generations.

Family stories are a crucial part of this legacy-building process. They not only help preserve the person's memory but also serve as a testament to the love and care that was given. By sharing these stories, caregivers can create lasting memories that honor the person they have lost while providing comfort and inspiration for others.

One such story is that of Sarah, who cared for her father in his final years. Despite the challenges of Alzheimer's, she found ways to connect with him and bring joy to his life. She would play his favorite music, read to him from his favorite books, and take him on walks in the park. Despite his memory loss, these activities brought his life a sense of peace and happiness. Sarah's story is not just a tale of caregiving but a testament to the power of love and its impact on a person's life.

But legacy-building isn't just about the past but also the future. Caregivers can use their experiences to educate and inspire others. They can share their stories, offer advice, and provide support to other families dealing with similar challenges. By doing so, they can create a legacy of hope and resilience that extends beyond their own lives.

One such inspirational tale is that of Mark, a caregiver for his mother with dementia. Despite the struggles, Mark found hope in unexpected places- in his mother's smile when she recognized him, in the laughter they shared during a favorite TV show, and in the quiet moments of connection amidst the confusion. His story serves as a beacon of hope for others facing similar challenges, reminding them that even in the darkest times, there can be moments of light.

Caregivers of Alzheimer's and dementia patients face an arduous task. Yet, amid the challenge and heartbreak, they are building a legacy of love, resilience, and care that will impact future generations. Their stories, filled with love and hope, remind us that even in the face of adversity, we can create something beautiful and lasting.

Building a legacy as a caregiver is not an easy task, but it's a worthwhile one. It allows you to honor your loved one in a profound way while also providing a source of inspiration and support for others. So, as you navigate the challenges of caregiving, remember that you are not just providing care—you are building a legacy.

A Call to Action

"The only thing necessary for the triumph of evil is for good men to do nothing."
- Edmund Burke.

This quote may seem out of place in our discussion about Alzheimer's and dementia, but its essence captures our purpose. As caregivers, family members, and concerned citizens, we must not stand idle in the face of these daunting conditions. It's time to raise our voices, increase awareness, and offer support.

Alzheimer's and dementia are battles fought every day by many around us.

But these battles often remain unseen and unheard to those not affected directly. It's our duty to bring these battles to light and share our stories, struggles, and victories. Each story shared is a beacon of hope, a testament to resilience, and a call for action.

Sharing your story and experiences with Alzheimer's and dementia can change the world. It can inspire others on a similar path, help them feel less alone, and provide insights they can apply in their own situations. Your story can spur research, create dialogues, and lead to new treatments or even a cure.

It's not just about sharing your own story, though. It's also about listening to the stories of others. Each story is a piece of a larger puzzle, a step towards a better understanding of these conditions. By sharing and listening, we can gather the knowledge and strength needed to face Alzheimer's and dementia head-on.

Beyond sharing, we must also take action. We need to support research efforts, advocate for better healthcare policies, and educate the public about Alzheimer's and dementia. We must strive for a world where these conditions are understood, not feared, and managed, not surrendered to. In this fight, we are not alone. There are countless organizations and groups dedicated to the cause. Find them, join them, and support them. Together, our voices are louder, our efforts more impactful.

Yet, taking action is about more than just the larger picture. It's also about the small, everyday acts of care and love. It's about being there for our loved ones, providing them with the best care possible, and creating moments of joy and connection.

Empowerment and resilience are our guiding lights in this journey. They are qualities we cultivate in ourselves and inspire in others. They give us the strength to face each new day, to meet each challenge, and to keep moving forward.

So, today, let's make a pledge. A pledge to share our stories, to listen to others, and to take action. A pledge to support those living with Alzheimer's and dementia and those caring for them. A pledge to empower and inspire, to show resilience in the face of adversity, and to keep hope alive.

This is our call to action, a call that echoes from every caregiver's heart, from every patient's struggle, and from every victory earned. It's a call for awareness, understanding, and support. It's a call for us to stand up, to speak out, and to make a difference.

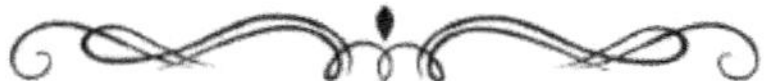

Chapter Eleven
Caregiver Health

"Taking care of yourself is part of taking care of others." - Author Unknown.

This quote is a gentle reminder that your health, as a caregiver, is vital. It's not just about the person you're caring for. It's about you too. You matter.

Caring for someone with Alzheimer's or dementia can be a challenge. It can drain you physically and emotionally. It's easy to forget about your own needs. But you can't pour from an empty cup. Your health is vital to providing quality care.

Your well-being also affects the person you're caring for. If you're stressed or tired, they may feel it, too. So, it's essential to take care of yourself. It's not selfish. It's necessary.

Eating right is an excellent place to start. Nutritious food gives you energy. It also boosts your immune system and helps you stay healthy. So, please eat well. Include fruits, vegetables, and lean proteins in your diet.
Exercise is also very important. It boosts your mood and energy levels and

helps you sleep better. Try to get at least thirty minutes of exercise each day. This could be a brisk walk or a yoga session. Do what works for you.

Taking breaks is healthy. It's okay to step away for a bit. It's okay to rest. You're human, not a machine. Taking breaks can refresh you and make you a better caregiver.

Sleep is also crucial for your health. Lack of sleep can make you feel tired and irritable. It can affect your ability to care for your loved one. So, try to get enough sleep. Make your bedroom a calm and quiet place. This can help you relax and sleep better.

Your mental health matters, too. Caring for someone with dementia can be stressful. It can be hard to see your loved one change. It's normal to feel sad or anxious. It's okay to ask for help. Reach out to a mental health professional if you need to.

Connecting with others can also help. You're not alone in this journey. Many people are going through the same thing. Join a support group. Talk to friends or family members. Share your feelings and experiences with them. It lightens your emotional load.

Taking care of yourself is not a luxury but a necessity. It's part of your role as a caregiver and is important for your loved one's well-being, too. So, make sure to take care of your health. You're worth it.

Caregiver Stress

"Caregiving often calls us to lean into love we didn't know possible." - Tia Walker.

Caregiving is a task that tests your strength. It's not easy. It takes physical, mental, and emotional tolls. When you care for someone with Alzheimer's or dementia, the stress can be high. You see your loved one change, lose memory, and struggle with daily tasks. This is difficult to watch. It's even harder to manage.

You might feel tired, sad, or angry. These feelings are normal. They prove your humanity. They show you care. But too much stress can be harmful. It's crucial to learn to manage this stress- your health matters. You can't care for others if you don't care for yourself first.

So, what can you do? Start by accepting your feelings. It's okay to feel upset or frustrated. It's okay to miss how things used to be. These feelings are valid, and they're part of the process. But don't let them consume you.

Remember, it's not your loved one's fault. Alzheimer's and dementia are diseases. They affect the brain in ways we don't fully understand. Your loved one is not choosing to forget. They're not purposely trying to make things difficult.

Next, find ways to relax. Take a walk, read a book, or meditate. You might find peace in nature, music, or art. Find what works for you. Make time for it each day. Even a few minutes can make a big difference.

It's also essential to stay healthy. Eat well, exercise, and get enough sleep. Your body needs good fuel to keep going. And don't forget to see your doctor regularly. Regular check-ups can catch any health issues early.

Reach out to others. Talk to friends or family about what you're going through. They might not fully understand, but they can offer support. They can lend an ear, a shoulder, or a hand when you need it.

You can also join a support group. There are many groups for caregivers of people with Alzheimer's or dementia. They offer a safe space to share your feelings, fears, and frustrations. You can learn from others who are in the same boat. You'll see you're not alone.

Don't try to do it all. It's okay to ask for help. You might need a break, or there might be tasks you can't handle alone. There are services out there that can help. Look for local resources.

Home health aides, adult day care centers, and respite care services exist. These can give you a break and provide care for your loved one. There's no shame in using these services. They're there to help.

You can also seek help from a therapist or counselor. They can offer strategies to cope with stress. They can provide a safe space to express your feelings. They can guide you to find balance in your life.

Caregiver Stress Check

"Taking care of yourself is part of taking care of others." - Jennifer Williamson.

Stress is a part and parcel of life, and you may find it amplified as a caregiver. The role of caregiver for someone with Alzheimer's or dementia is a tough one. It is filled with emotional ups and downs, physical demands, and mental challenges. This section aims to help you check and manage your stress levels.

The first step in managing stress is recognizing it. It can manifest in various ways - you may feel tired all the time, or you may find yourself getting annoyed quickly. You might have trouble sleeping or lack interest in things you used to enjoy. These are all signs of stress and burnout that you should take seriously.

Next, it's essential to understand that feeling stressed is okay. You're dealing with a complex situation. It's normal to feel overwhelmed. Don't be hard on yourself for feeling this way. Instead, focus on ways to manage this stress and take care of yourself.

One effective method to manage stress is to take regular breaks. Even a few minutes away can help. You could go for a short walk, read a few pages of a book, or just sit quietly in a room. These breaks can help clear your mind and relieve some of the tension.

Another way is to get regular exercise. It can be as simple as a daily walk or as structured as a yoga class. Exercise not only helps keep you in good health but also releases chemicals in your brain that can improve your mood and reduce stress levels.

Eating a balanced diet is also vital. Proper nutrition can boost your energy levels and keep your body functioning at its best. Try to incorporate fresh fruits, vegetables, lean proteins, and whole grains into your meals.

Sleep is another crucial factor. A lack of sleep can amplify feelings of stress and make it harder to cope. Try to establish a regular sleep schedule and create a relaxing bedtime routine to help you get the rest you need.

It's also beneficial to talk about your feelings. This could be with a friend, family member, or a support group. Sharing your experiences can help relieve some of the burden and make you feel less alone.

Lastly, remember to make time for things you enjoy. It's easy to get caught up in caregiving duties and forget about your own needs and interests. But making time for hobbies or activities you love can significantly reduce stress.

Caregiver Depression

"Caring for the mind is as crucial and challenging as taking care of the body. In fact, one cannot be healthy without the other." - Sid Garza-Hillman.

Being a caregiver for a loved one with Alzheimer's or dementia is challenging. It can take a toll on your health, including your mental health. One common issue caregivers face is depression.

Depression is not just feeling sad. It's a medical condition. It can impact every part of your life. It can make you feel tired all the time. It can make it hard to focus. It can even lead to physical health issues.

Not all caregivers will get depression. But many do. It's a heavy load to bear. You are not alone if you feel this way. There are ways to manage and treat depression.

First, you need to know the signs. Depression is more than just a low mood. It can cause a loss of interest in things you used to enjoy. It can disturb your sleep. It can change your appetite. It can make you feel worthless or guilty.

Knowing these signs is helpful. Recognizing your depression early and seeking treatment can make a huge difference.

Next, don't be afraid to seek help. Mental health is important. It's just as important as physical health. Don't ignore the signs of depression. Don't try to "tough it out." If you're feeling depressed, reach out to a health professional.

There are many treatments for depression, including therapy and medication. These treatments can help manage your symptoms. They can improve your quality of life. Reach out if you are struggling and seek help.

Grief and Loss as Alzheimer's Progresses

"Grief is like the ocean; it comes in waves, ebbing and flowing. Sometimes the water is calm, and sometimes it is overwhelming. All we can do is learn to swim."
- Vicki Harrison.

As Alzheimer's progresses, you, as a caregiver, may experience a type of grief called anticipatory grief. It's a feeling of loss before a death or dreaded event occurs. In the case of Alzheimer's, it is the gradual loss of the person you once knew. The person is still there, but their memory and cognitive abilities are slowly fading away.

This can be, without a doubt, a tough time. But know that it's okay to grieve. It's okay to feel sorrow for the changes in your loved one and the relationship you had with them. It's a natural response to what you're going through.

The first step towards dealing with this grief is acceptance. Acceptance doesn't mean you're okay with the situation, but it's understanding that it's happening and you can't change it. It's accepting that your loved one is changing and the relationship you had is evolving.

Next, seek support. You don't have to go through this journey alone. Reach out to friends, family, or a support group. Many are going through the same experience, and their support can be invaluable.

Also, keep in mind that it's okay to feel joy. Your loved one may not remember past events, but they can still experience happiness in the moment. So, create new joyful moments with them.

Be patient with yourself. Grief is not linear; it comes in waves. Some days will be harder than others. On those tough days, remind yourself that it's okay to feel the way you do. Allow yourself to feel the sadness, but also remember your love for your loved one.

Understanding and acknowledging your grief can be a powerful tool in your caregiving journey. By recognizing your feelings of loss, seeking support, and taking care of your emotional health, you can navigate this challenging time with resilience and grace.

Chapter Twelve
Breaking Ground: Insights from the Newest Research

"Research means that you don't know, but are willing to find out." - Charles F. Kettering.

Since the initial creation of this book, numerous recent studies have emerged, bringing forth novel information and groundbreaking developments in the realm of Alzheimer's and dementia. As we've consistently emphasized, knowledge holds significant power, and continuous understanding is vital in staying abreast of the latest advancements in this field.

Dementia Among Younger People Linked to 15 Factors

In recent years, there has been a noticeable increase in early-onset dementia, and a comprehensive new study conducted by researchers from Maastricht University (UM) in the Netherlands and the University of Exeter in the U.K. has pinpointed the likely causes. Published on December 26, 2023, in JAMA Neurology, the study identifies 15 factors associated with the onset of dementia at a younger age.

Drawing on data from the UK Biobank, encompassing 356,052 participants aged 65 and younger without a prior dementia diagnosis, the study reveals a range of factors contributing to early-onset dementia. These include:

1. Lower formal education
2. Lower socioeconomic status
3. The presence of the apolipoprotein ε4 allele (APOE ε4 – a significant genetic risk factor for Alzheimer's disease)
4. Complete abstinence from alcohol
5. Alcohol use disorder
6. Social isolation
7. Vitamin D deficiency
8. Elevated levels of C-reactive protein (indicative of increased inflammation)
9. Reduced handgrip strength
10. Hearing impairment
11. Orthostatic hypotension
12. History of stroke
13. Diabetes
14. Heart disease
15. Depression

One surprising revelation from the study concerns alcohol-related findings. Contrary to expectations, both moderate and heavy alcohol users exhibited a lower risk of young-onset dementia compared to those who abstained from alcohol entirely.

Young-onset dementia, characterized by cognitive decline occurring before the age of 65, affects approximately 370,000 individuals each year, as noted in a press release from MU. The study underscores the importance of early diagnosis and support for those with young-onset dementia.

Given the limited research on risk factors for young-onset dementia, this new study stands as a valuable and much-welcomed addition to our understanding of this complex condition.

New Alzheimer's Treatment Accelerates Removal of Plaque from the Brain

In the initial clinical human trials, a promising new Alzheimer's therapy has exhibited potential, marking a significant breakthrough. Researchers at the West Virginia University Rockefeller Neuroscience Institute (RNI) discovered that the combination of focused ultrasound and antibody therapies could accelerate the removal of amyloid-beta plaques from the brains of individuals with Alzheimer's disease.

Published in The New England Journal of Medicine on January 11, 2024 the study showcases the positive outcomes of this innovative approach. Amyloid-beta plaques, characterized by an abnormal buildup of proteins, are a distinctive feature of Alzheimer's. These proteins tend to clump together, forming plaques that disrupt normal neuronal function in the brain.

Monoclonal antibody treatments targeting amyloid-beta, including aducanumab and lecanemab, have proven effective in clearing these plaques and slowing down the progression of the disease. The integration of focused ultrasound with these antibody therapies, as explored by the RNI researchers, presents a promising avenue for advancing Alzheimer's treatment.

Fasting Could Reduce Signs of Alzheimer's Disease

Other studies show that Mice that ate on a time-restricted schedule showed memory improvements and fewer signs of dementia. Engaging in intermittent (time-restricted) fasting may contribute to a decreased risk of cognitive deterioration, as per a recent study featured in the journal Cell Metabolism.

Scientists at the University of California San Diego School of Medicine modified the feeding regimen of specific groups of mice, restricting their eating to six-hour windows each day.

New Blood Test to Detect Alzheimer's

A potential breakthrough in the early detection of Alzheimer's disease has been reported by researchers. According to a recent study, a simple blood test may be able to identify the presence of the disease before symptoms manifest, offering a more affordable and less invasive alternative to brain scans and lumbar punctures.

The study, published in JAMA Neurology focused on testing blood for a protein called p-tau217, a crucial biomarker for Alzheimer's. This protein's levels increase simultaneously with other Alzheimer's-related proteins, allowing for early detection. The accuracy of identifying increased levels of beta amyloid was found to be up to 96%, while detecting tau was 97% accurate through testing for p-tau217, making it a promising and accessible diagnostic method. This development aligns with ongoing efforts to make Alzheimer's tests more cost-effective and widely available, coinciding with advancements in potential drugs that could slow the disease's progression.

The Power of Play for Dementia Patients

There is more research to be done. But researchers are finding that thinking with your hands and leaving your brain out of the equation is helpful with all dementia patients. Pioneers in using LEGO bricks for older folks and their caregivers note the potential for unlocking memories, engaging the mind, and staying calm.

Other Helpful Resources

- Dementia Guidance - https://www.waughconsulting.info/
- Clinical trials for Alzheimer's and Dementia - https://clinicaltrials.gov
- National Institute on Aging - https://www.nia.nih.gov/
- British Medical Journal on Alzheimer's - https://www.bmj.com/content/338/bmj.b158

My friends, there is more research to be done. But current data is showing that there is hope on the horizon to prevent and help treat

Alzheimers and dementia.

Conclusion

"The secret of change is to focus all of your energy, not on fighting the old, but on building the new." - Socrates.

As we reflect on our journey through the landscape of Alzheimer's and dementia, we find ourselves returning to the key takeaways from each chapter. These insights, like beacons in the fog, guide us through the complex terrain of caregiving. They remind us of the importance of understanding, caregiving, and emotional support in our role as caregivers. Let's take a moment to revisit these pivotal points.

In the early stages of this journey, we sought to understand the mechanics of Alzheimer's and dementia. We learned about the causes, symptoms, and progression of these conditions. This knowledge equipped us with the tools we need to navigate the road ahead. Understanding is the first step to empowerment. And with this understanding, we can provide more effective care for our loved ones.

As we delved deeper into the subject, we explored the art and science of caregiving. We learned about the importance of routines, the value of patience, and the power of empathy. These caregiving strategies not only improve the quality of life for our loved ones but also enhance our own well-being. Through caregiving, we become a beacon of hope and light in their lives.

At the heart of our journey lies emotional support. We learned about the power of empathy, compassion, and love in the face of Alzheimer's and dementia. These virtues not only support our loved ones but also nourish our own spirits. They remind us that we are not alone in this journey. Through emotional support, we strengthen the bonds that hold us together in the face of adversity.

Throughout this book, we've learned that understanding, caregiving, and emotional support are not just skills to be mastered. They are also forms of empowerment. They enable us to rise above the challenges of Alzheimer's and dementia, transforming us from mere caregivers into champions of love and resilience. This transformation is not easy, but it is undeniably rewarding.

As we come to the end of this book, let us not forget the power of hope. Hope is the light that guides us through the darkest nights. It is the spark that ignites our courage, fuels our resilience, and empowers us to face the challenges of Alzheimer's and dementia. And as long as we have hope, we can navigate any storm.

In closing, let's remember that our journey doesn't end here. The road to understanding, caregiving, and emotional support is a lifelong journey. It is a journey marked by growth, resilience, and love. And as we continue this journey, let's carry with us the lessons we've learned, the insights we've gained, and the hope we've kindled.

The purpose of this book was to empower you, the caregiver, to provide the best possible care for your loved one with Alzheimer's or dementia. By understanding these conditions, improving your caregiving skills, and enhancing emotional support, you can significantly improve the quality of life for both you and your loved one. Remember, you are not alone on this journey, and you are more powerful than you think. Keep learning, keep loving, and keep hoping. Your journey continues; every step you take is a testament to your strength, resilience, and love.

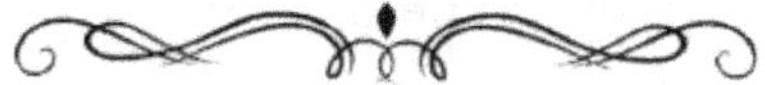

References

Books

Kitwood, T. (1997). *Dementia Reconsidered: The Person Comes First*. Open University Press.

Post, S. G. (2000). *The Moral Challenge of Alzheimer Disease*. Johns Hopkins University Press.

Mace, N. L., & Rabins, P. V. (2011). *The 36-Hour Day: A Family Guide to Caring for People Who Have Alzheimer Disease*. Johns Hopkins University Press.

Power, G. A. (2010). *Dementia Beyond Drugs: Changing the Culture of Care*. Health Professions Press.

James, O. (2014). *Contented Dementia*. Vermilion.

Snow, L. (2008). *Speaking Dementia: Making Sense Of It All*. New Dawn Press.

Gwyther, L. P., & Whitehouse, P. J. (2001). *Coping with Alzheimer's: A Caregiver's Emotional Survival Guide*. Rodale Books.

Zgola, J. (1999). *Care That Works: A Relationship Approach to Persons with*

Dementia. Johns Hopkins University Press.

Norberg, K., & Graff, M. J. (2008). *Caring for a Loved One with Alzheimer's: An Emotional Journey*. Prometheus Books.

Schall, M. L. (2000). *A Caregiver's Guide to Alzheimer's Disease: 300 Tips for Making Life Easier*. Demos Medical Publishing.

Journals

Perry, E. K., & Perry, R. H. (1993). "Neurotransmitter and Neuropathological Changes in Alzheimer's Disease." *Journal of Neurology, Neurosurgery, and Psychiatry, 56*(7), 735-741.

Kitwood, T. (1997). "The Experience of Dementia." *Aging & Mental Health, 1*(1), 13-22.

Ballard, C., O'Brien, J., & James, I. (2001). "Dementia: Management of Behavioural and Psychological Symptoms." *Oxford University Press, 59*(5), 575-583.

Brodaty, H., & Donkin, M. (2009). "Family Caregivers of People with Dementia." *Dialogues in Clinical Neuroscience, 11*(2), 217-228.

Cohen, D., & Eisdorfer, C. (1986). "The Loss of Self: A Family Resource for the Care of Alzheimer's Disease and Related Disorders." *The Gerontologist, 26*(5), 531-538.

Galvin, J. E., & Sadowsky, C. H. (2012). "Practical Guidelines for the Recognition and Diagnosis of Dementia." *Journal of the American Board of Family Medicine, 25*(3), 367-382.

Graham, J. E., Rockwood, K., & Beattie, B. L. (1997). "Prevalence and Severity of Cognitive Impairment with and without Dementia in an Elderly Population." *Lancet, 349*(9068), 1793-1796.

Kitwood, T., & Bredin, K. (1992). "Towards a Theory of Dementia Care: Personhood and Well-being." *Ageing and Society, 12*(3), 269-287.

Mittelman, M. S., Ferris, S. H., Shulman, E., Steinberg, G., & Levin, B. (1996). "A Family Intervention to Delay Nursing Home Placement of Patients with Alzheimer Disease." *Journal of the American Medical Association, 276*(21), 1725-1731.

Schulz, R., & Martire, L. M. (2004). "Family Caregiving of Persons with Dementia: Prevalence, Health Effects, and Support Strategies." *The American Journal of Geriatric Psychiatry, 12*(3), 240-249.

Web Articles

Alzheimer's Association. (2023). "Alzheimer's Disease Facts and Figures." Retrieved from [Alzheimer's Association website].

Mayo Clinic. (2023). "Alzheimer's Treatments: What's on the Horizon?" Retrieved from [Mayo Clinic website].

National Institute on Aging. (2023). "Caring for a Person with Alzheimer's Disease." Retrieved from [NIA website].

AARP. (2023). "10 Warning Signs of Alzheimer's." Retrieved from [AARP website].

WebMD. (2023). "Understanding Alzheimer's Disease: the Basics." Retrieved from [WebMD website].

Caregiver.org. (2023). "Caregiver's Guide to Understanding Dementia Behaviors." Retrieved from [Caregiver.org website].

Healthline. (2023). "Living with Dementia: Tips and Resources." Retrieved from [Healthline website].

Dementia.org. (2023). "Stages of Dementia: Understanding

Progression." Retrieved from [Dementia.org website].

Alzheimer's Society. (2023). "Legal and Financial Planning for Alzheimer's Disease." Retrieved from [Alzheimer's Society website].

CDC. (2023). "Alzheimer's Disease and Healthy Aging." Retrieved from CDC website].

Gupta, S (November 03, 2022). "The 7 Stages of Dementia: What to Expect" verywellmind. https://www.verywellmind.com/the-7-stages-of-dementia-symptoms-and-what-to-expect-6823696.

Rudy, M (January 10, 2024). "Dementia Among Younger People is Linked to 15 Factors, Major Study Reveals." Fox News. https://www.foxnews.com/health/dementia-younger-people-linked-15-factors-major-study-reveals.

Rudy, M (July 18, 2023). "New dementia drug 'has given me hope': Alzheimer's patients reveal their stories." Fox News. https://www.foxnews.com/health/dementia-drug-given-me-hope-alzheimers-patients-reveal-stories.

Rudy, M (July 18, 2023). "Fasting could reduce signs of Alzheimer's disease, studies suggest: 'Profound effects'" Fox News. https://www.foxnews.com/health/fasting-could-reduce-signs-alzheimers-disease-studies-suggest-profound-effects.

The National Desk (January 26, 2024). "New blood test could be game-changer for detecting Alzheimer's." KATU2ABC. https://katu.com/news/nation-world/new-blood-test-could-be-game-changer-for-detecting-alzheimers-ptau217-dementia-proteins-biomarkers-alzpath-beta-amyloid-tau.

Denney, Amy (January 29, 2024). "The Power of Play for Dementia Patients." The Epoch Times. https://www.theepochtimes.com/health/the-power-of-play-for-dementia-patients-5569442.

www.ingramcontent.com/pod-product-compliance
Lightning Source LLC
Chambersburg PA
CBHW071747150726
47998CB00005B/1845